The
Collective
Cure

UPSTREAM SOLUTIONS
FOR BETTER
PUBLIC HEALTH

MONICA L. WANG

BEACON PRESS, BOSTON

BEACON PRESS
24 Farnsworth Street
Boston, Massachusetts
www.beacon.org

Beacon Press books
are published under the auspices of
the Unitarian Universalist Association of Congregations.

29 28 27 26   8 7 6 5 4 3 2 1

This book is printed on acid-free paper that meets the uncoated paper
ANSI/NISO specifications for permanence as revised in 1992.

Text design and composition by Kim Arney

All stories in this book are based on true events and have been
carefully validated through interviews, confirmation with participants,
and cross-referencing. To respect privacy, some names and
identifying details have been changed.

Library of Congress Cataloging-in-Publication Data is available for this title.
ISBN: 978-0-8070-1749-4; e-book: 978-0-8070-1750-0;
audiobook: 978-0-8070-2295-5

The authorized representative in the EU for product safety and
compliance is Easy Access System Europe 16879218, Mustamäe tee 50,
10621 Tallinn, Estonia: http://beacon.org/eu-contact.

To my parents,
whose hard work and sacrifices
paved the way for a better life for me.

To my husband,
for dreaming big and bold with me
and believing in a future where
we can make a difference.

To my children,
who inspire me daily to work toward
building a world where health and
opportunity are not defined by
the circumstances of birth.
May you, and millions of others,
live and thrive in a world
that champions well-being for all.

Contents

Introduction

On Sunday, May 5, 2013, I walked into a windowless classroom on the ground floor level of the FXB Building at the Harvard T. H. Chan School of Public Health. The building was quiet, as expected for a weekend, but two classrooms were alive with the buzz of physicians attending their weekend sessions in a part-time graduate program.

At twenty-eight, I was just one year past earning my doctorate from that same institution and in the midst of a postdoctoral fellowship at the University of Massachusetts Medical School in preventive and behavioral medicine. Professor Nancy Kane, a respected leader in health care policy and education, had recently recruited me to develop and teach a hybrid course (part online, part in person) for mid-career physicians in Harvard's Master in Health Care Management (MHCM) program. This executive part-time program is designed to hone the leadership skills of physician professionals shaping the future of health care.

Students in this program weren't the typical graduate students I had taught in the master of public health (MPH) program. They were seasoned physicians, most in their forties or fifties, carving out time from the demands of their medical careers to gain leadership and management skills as they advanced in health care. Many were already established attending physicians or held management roles, balancing clinical responsibilities and career ambitions with family lives that included spouses and children. I was two years into married life, without children of my own yet, and just beginning my career.

On that warm spring day, I was about to meet my first cohort, introducing myself as their instructor and presenting the new course I'd designed to guide them through the social determinants of health—a topic I was deeply passionate about and one that Nancy Kane and I believed was vital for them to understand as current and future health care leaders. I entered the room and found myself looking out at rows of mostly white, mostly male faces—many at least two decades older than I was at the time. A few students nodded or smiled, but most stared back with thinly veiled doubt.

A peculiar sight it must have been: a classroom full of experienced physicians, with a younger, immigrant, Chinese American woman who was newly minted in public health, not in medicine or management, as their instructor. I was the opposite of what many were accustomed to seeing standing at the front of a room: non-male, non-white, non-physician, and decidedly non-tall.

Stop. Center yourself. I had a doctorate and a master's in public health from Harvard. I brought academic expertise and lived experience to this material, and I was deeply passionate about sharing it. I was bold, driven, curious, and creative in finding solutions. And I believed I had something valuable to offer—whether or not it fit the package others were expecting.

I took a breath and began, introducing myself and diving into the course's format and objectives. Barely a minute in, a male physician to my far left in the front row, red faced and fist raised, interrupted.

"Have you taught before?" he demanded, his voice sharp with challenge. I watched the pink flush spread across his cheeks and heard the murmurs rippling through the room.

"Yes, I have," I replied evenly, holding his gaze. "Not in this program, but I've taught other graduate courses here at Harvard."

My voice was steady, though I could feel the heat climbing up my neck. *Observe it, don't absorb it.* I wasn't there to teach them surgery; I was there to teach what I know.

Another male physician, seated in a center row, leaned forward, eyes locked on mine. "We're going to be tough on you."

"I wouldn't expect anything less," I replied, sensing he was giving me a direct, if public, warning.

It was clear that at least some of the students weren't thrilled about the situation—whether it was about taking a course on a topic they might not have considered useful in a health care management program, having a much younger instructor, having a hybrid course format (which, at the time, was still unconventional), or a combination of all three. To be fair, if I were in their shoes, I might have felt skeptical too. But I knew myself better than they did and believed in what I could bring to the table. Still, a small seed of doubt crept in. Had I made a mistake by signing up to teach in this program?

After I had finished the course introduction and went back to my research, I reminded myself of Nancy's faith in me. As the cofounder and director of the MHCM program and a respected senior faculty member, her opinion carried significant weight. She had seen me teach the material to Harvard graduate students before, and I didn't believe she would have brought me into the program if she didn't think I was up to the challenge.

I had poured hundreds of hours into developing the online modules, which were based on Dr. Ichiro Kawachi's Society and Health course. His pioneering research in social determinants had been pivotal in shaping my understanding of how social conditions impact health. This course wasn't just about the history and research behind disease prevention; it was about presenting a broader vision of health and well-being, one that acknowledges the social and structural forces shaping people's lives long before they see a doctor. This vision was shaped by the many thought leaders and professors who deepened my understanding during my graduate training and beyond, including Drs. Ichiro Kawachi, David Williams, Nancy Krieger, Marie McCormick, Camara Jones, Arline Geronimus, and many others. Their groundbreaking work laid the foundation for addressing health from every angle. Their contributions continue to drive the field forward, highlighting how each of our lives is shaped by social and structural determinants.

The Collective Cure is about understanding these powerful forces and recognizing the role we can each play—however small or large—in building healthier communities. It is both a tribute to and a call to action for better health for all, a vision that reaches beyond the walls of public health and medicine to touch each of us. Through compelling personal stories, we'll explore how factors like family income, race and ethnicity, the neighborhoods we live in, our work environments, and our social connections all shape our health. Together, we'll move from understanding these determinants to finding actionable solutions that improve health for all.

In these pages, you'll see the data and science behind social determinants of health come to life through the stories of women I interviewed firsthand. These stories illustrated how long-standing social and structural factors shaped health long before public health crises like the COVID-19 pandemic, and how the pandemic worsened these disparities. You'll meet Marielis Rosa, a first-generation college student navigating remote learning from Section 8 housing in New York City during the pandemic, revealing the toll that economic and educational barriers take on health and the lifeline that social connections can offer. In Panola, Alabama, you'll learn about Dorothy Oliver, who worked tirelessly to safeguard her predominantly Black community, highlighting the profound lack of infrastructure and broadband access in rural areas—challenges that the pandemic only made more urgent. In Manchaca, Texas, we'll explore how Indigenous social worker Rosa Tupina Yaotonalcuauhtli fought to preserve Mexica Indigenous knowledge and culture, as the pandemic's erosion of these practices deepened historical trauma and exacerbated health inequities.

Interwoven with their stories is my own, as I navigate social determinants of health both professionally and personally. As a Chinese American woman born in Wuhan, I watched the pandemic unfold, balancing my role as a public health expert with the experience of being an Asian American during a time of heightened xenophobia. The crisis reshaped public health and intensified racial and cultural challenges I had long faced.

Growing up as a student in Boston's school desegregation program, I was one of a small group of students of color who lived in the city but attended school in a predominantly white suburb. This experience deepened my understanding of structural and systemic racism, highlighting its lasting impact on neighborhood disparities and health. Later, as a full-time professor and mother of two young children during the pandemic, I experienced firsthand the toll of job stress on mental and physical health, while also grappling with the gender inequalities that many working mothers and caregivers face. These experiences have strengthened my conviction that addressing health inequities requires comprehensive solutions that tackle both the visible and invisible barriers to well-being, creating a world where opportunities for good health are the default, not the exception.

To truly improve health, we cannot simply focus on treating people once illness or crisis takes hold. Downstream interventions like medical treatments, surgeries, and urgent care are essential, but they cannot address the root causes of health and disease. It's like putting a Band-Aid on a deep wound or trying to rescue people after they've already fallen into a stormy river. To create lasting change, we must move upstream, tackling the systems and structures that shape health long before illness strikes.

Later that day over dinner, I recounted the physician students' "meet and greet" to my husband Luke, who at the time was in his first year of medical school. By that point, my level of enthusiasm for teaching the course probably matched the students' for having to take it.

"Yes, they are going to be hard on you, and you need to be ready for it," he responded, sensing the challenge ahead. "But remember, you don't need to reach all of them. If you reach just one or two with the material, you'll have made a difference."

He was right. I couldn't control how they digested the material, their actions and reactions—or anyone else's, for that matter. What I could control was how I showed up and whether I gave my very best on a topic and a field I believe are essential to health care and our society, one that fills the pages of this book.

Here we go.

CHAPTER I

The Myth of
the Great Equalizer

From as early as I can remember, the story my parents told me was the same: anyone, no matter how little or how much they had, could create a better future if they worked hard enough at their studies. It was a story wrapped in hope, a simple, almost magical promise that education would be the key to unlocking a future of possibility.

For our family, this promise had a clear path: get good grades, score well on exams, go to college, pursue an advanced degree, and land a respectable, well-paying job in a field like medicine or law. Failure, in this story, was never an option. It was a belief deeply ingrained in our family ethos and in American society at large. After all, this was the crux of the American Dream: anyone, regardless of the circumstances they were born into, could chart a course toward success through hard work and education as the great equalizer.

This was the dream that my dad had brought to life. Both he and my mother grew up in food-insecure households, raised by working-class parents in a time of significant social and economic upheaval in China in the late 1950s and '60s. Despite working long days, both sets of my grandparents struggled to put food on the table. My dad, the youngest of five, and my mom, the oldest of four, often went hungry. Photos from their teenage and early adult years show them to be painfully thin.

"Sometimes, all we got for dinner growing up was a mouthful of rice," my mom would often say when I was child, chiding me for leaving food on my plate. "Finish your food."

As a young student in Wuhan, my father excelled in his studies from elementary school through university, particularly in English, an area in which he was exceptional. This wasn't just a source of pride for him or his family; it represented a chance for a better life. When a visiting professor from the US recognized his talent, he encouraged my dad to apply to graduate school in Boston. He was accepted into the language arts PhD program at Boston University, earning a full scholarship and a modest stipend. To Boston he went, living largely off ramen noodles and working as a dishwasher to earn extra money.

He spent much of his paycheck to improve my grandparents' quality of life back home, buying them modern essentials like a refrigerator, washing machine, TV, and even a camcorder (for those of you born after the 1990s, that's a pre-smartphone video recorder). Slowly but surely, he climbed the social and economic ladder. With his doctorate in hand, he secured a full-time faculty position, and by the time I was almost four, he had saved enough to bring my mother and me to the US. He knew that America offered more opportunities to build a wealthier—and healthier—life.

Indeed, our family in the US has greater economic resources than my family back in Wuhan. Immigrating here has given us more opportunities to have stable jobs, private health insurance through our employers, access to quality health care, nutritious food, safe housing, and cleaner air. My parents, my brother, and I enjoy overall good health, with few to no chronic conditions. We have the freedom to go to work, travel, pursue hobbies, and connect with family, friends, and colleagues. Still a full-time academic, my dad continues to shovel the heavy New England snow in winter, mow the lawn under the summer sun, and chase after his granddaughters, never slowing down. My mother continues to work full-time as a nurse aide and is on her feet most of the day. She carries heavy grocery bags up the stairs without breaking a sweat, tends to her garden with pride, and delights in sending us pictures of vegetables as they're harvested.

Yet, the contrast between my family's experience and that of my relatives back in China is stark. Despite having similar genetics, many of our relatives in China suffer from chronic conditions like hypertension, heart disease, and cancer. All four of my grandparents have passed away prematurely due to cancer, dementia, or other chronic illnesses. As I think about the journey my family has made—from food insecurity and poor health to stability—I'm reminded of the many others for whom the same path isn't so straightforward.

Take, for example, Marielis Rosa, a first-generation Latina freshman at Boston University. At eighteen years old, she faced a different kind of hardship, one that reflected the economic realities of being a low-income student, the systemic challenges of socioeconomic health disparities, and the rapid disruption of the COVID-19 pandemic.

In March 2020, while I was preparing another research grant proposal, Marielis was sitting at her family's tiny kitchen table in Brooklyn, planning to pick up shifts at a local children's recreational center to pay for her student fees.[1] There, she opened an email from Boston University: "We strongly advise that students who are not presently on campus do not return to campus at the conclusion of spring break." As the virus spread rapidly across the US and around the world, colleges and universities were shutting down, banning students from returning.

Like millions of students, Marielis's immediate reactions were shock and dismay, though perhaps for reasons different from many of her peers. She grew up in a cramped Section 8 apartment in Brooklyn, where space was scarce and sunlight even scarcer. Her small bedroom had a single, narrow window that let in only slivers of light, often blocked by the neighboring building. When she arrived at Boston University, her dorm room felt like a sanctuary. Four expansive windows flooded the space with natural light and offered sweeping views of the city. It wasn't just the sunlight or the view. The dorm provided reliable heat, hot water, stable internet access, and, for the first time, a private space she could truly call her own. For her, college wasn't just a place to study, sleep, and socialize; it was a refuge where she could focus, dream, and feel safe.

With the first semester under her belt, she had been eager to explore her new campus, make connections, and dive deeper into her coursework in political science and sociology. But as the gravity of the situation set in, Marielis quickly brushed aside her disappointment, feeling selfish. There was nothing to do but do what she had always done: find a way to get through the day, week, month, and year, and help her family do the same.

She called a cousin, the only family member she knew with a car, to help pack her dorm belongings and drive her back to Brooklyn. Initially, she stayed with her mom in her old childhood apartment, but soon after, she moved in with her sister (who also lived in Section 8 housing) to help care for her sister's two children: a twelve-year-old son and a six-year-old daughter.

With her sister as the only working adult in the household, serving as a frontline administrative staff member covering long shifts in the ER, Marielis took on the responsibility of caring for her nephew and niece during the day while managing her remote coursework and exams. The days seemed to blend in an endless carousel of tasks: prepare food, tidy up, keep children entertained or occupied, and start the cycle anew. She paid attention as best she could to her class Zoom lectures, and the bulk of her work took place in the evening when her sister returned home.

Despite the unexpected challenges, Marielis remained steadfast in her determination to succeed academically. Late nights were spent hunched over used textbooks and online articles, the dim glow of her laptop, set to the lowest brightness to save battery, illuminating her tired yet focused face. She was the first in her family to apply and get accepted into college—a milestone that had proved far more challenging to navigate than she had anticipated. Her family did not have the knowledge or resources to help guide her through the application process of essays, fees, and deadlines. Every step forward required careful consideration and trade-offs: How many schools could she afford to apply to? Which universities offered scholarships she was eligible for and were close enough to home in case of emergency? How much of her high school part-time job earnings should she spend on application fees versus saving for other expenses like a laptop, toiletries, and a suitcase?

A degree from college was a crucial step to climbing the social and economic ladder to a better life. Every dollar spent was an investment in her future, a small sacrifice in pursuit of a brighter tomorrow. Right?

The research paints a clear picture: educational attainment is consistently linked with better health and longer lifespan.[2] For many, a college degree is a pathway to greater job opportunities and lifetime earnings—factors that directly contribute to improved health.[3] Studies show a clear pattern in average salary by education level; with each step up the educational ladder, people can generally expect to earn a higher living wage.[4] People with higher levels of education are more likely to secure higher-paying, stable jobs with benefits and enjoy better access to health care, all of which are closely linked with improved health.[5]

Furthermore, higher education is strongly linked with higher *socioeconomic status* (SES), an individual's position in a social hierarchy based on prestige and access to resources.[6] Higher levels of education elevate SES through higher income, more prestigious occupations, and increased opportunity to build wealth. This increased wealth and status open the door to essential health-promoting resources, including nutritious food, safe housing, quality health care, and living in a healthy neighborhood.[7] It also facilitates access to other crucial resources, such as supportive social networks, reliable transportation, and modern technology.

Research also highlights the positive impact of education on mental health. Higher levels of education are associated with lower levels of stress, depression, and anxiety, along with improved coping skills and stronger social support networks that protect against life's stressors.[8] Education can also promote healthier behaviors; higher levels of education are linked with lower rates of smoking and alcohol consumption, higher levels of physical activity, and better quality diets.[9] Additionally, education improves health literacy (the ability to obtain, understand, and use health information to make informed decisions). Individuals with health literacy can better navigate the health care system, communicate more effectively with health care professionals, advocate for their health needs, seek timely medical care, and follow treatment plans.[10]

Ample research points to the *socioeconomic health gradient*, a clear pattern showing that individuals in higher SES groups generally experience better health than those in lower SES groups.[11] Large-scale studies and meta-analyses consistently show that this pattern holds true across different time periods, demographic groups (including gender, race, ethnicity, and country),[12] child and adult populations,[13] and most measures of health and disease,[14] including premature mortality.[15] Whether we're talking about infectious diseases like COVID or chronic diseases like cancer, the story remains the same: those with higher education levels and higher SES generally live longer, healthier lives.

This gradient holds true for people of all racial and ethnic backgrounds. In a 2006 landmark study,[16] researchers compared the health of adults in the US and England, considering factors like income, education, age, and health behaviors. Because race and ethnicity are also linked with health (which we will unpack in depth in the next few chapters), the researchers looked at data from non-Hispanic/Latino white adults *only*. The results showed two key findings: White Americans were generally less healthy than their white British counterparts, with higher rates of chronic diseases like diabetes and heart disease. And in both countries, among white adults, lower levels of income and education predicted higher rates of disease. Remarkably, these patterns remained significant even after adjusting for common behavioral risk factors like smoking, obesity, and alcohol consumption.

Studies like this challenge the assumption that race is the primary factor in determining health, reminding us that socioeconomic disparities in health often outweigh racial disparities. By recognizing the socioeconomic health gradient within and across all racial groups, we can shift our focus to the broader social and economic context that shapes everyone's lives. After all, the gradient emphasizes that access to resources, such as quality education, stable employment, safe housing, and health care, has a greater impact on health than race or ethnicity alone.

Decades of scientific evidence highlight the link between SES and health across the globe. Stories like my dad's remain the exception rather than the rule. This raises the question: How can one factor equalize when all else is not equal? While education plays a pivotal role in shaping health and opportunity, it is not sufficient on its own to ensure good health. The reality is far more nuanced, and determinants of health other than education are extremely powerful. Structural determinants like economic inequality and limited access to resources continue to present significant barriers to opportunity and well-being, regardless of how hard individuals like Marielis or my dad work.

While *social determinants of health* refer to the social, economic, and environmental factors that influence health,[17] *structural determinants of health* are the broader societal and institutional forces that shape these factors and perpetuate health inequities on a population level.[18] In Marielis's case, a college degree is a social determinant of health, whereas the limited educational resources and support systems for first-generation, low-income students like her are a structural determinant of health. Other structural barriers that make it harder for students like Marielis to climb the education ladder include high tuition costs and limited access to financial aid.[19] There was no college savings account set aside for Marielis or my dad, no parental support for textbooks, fees, and living expenses. Without scholarships, neither one of them would have been able to attend university.

Students in low-income neighborhoods are also more likely to experience structural disparities in the quality of K–12 education. They often have less access to experienced teachers, advanced coursework, and extracurricular activities, which can hinder their academic preparation and competitiveness for higher education.[20] Institutional policies, such as complex application processes, legacy admissions, standardized testing requirements, and the availability of support services like counseling, tutoring, and essay writing, can either facilitate or impede access to higher education, depending on whether families can navigate and afford to give their children a leg up.[21] Finally, early-life social and economic factors such as family income, parental education level, and neighborhood resources also influence one's ability to pursue higher education.[22] These structural inequities (systemic disparities in access to resources, opportunities, and outcomes based on factors like socioeconomic status, gender, race, ethnicity, and other aspects of identity) create multiple barriers for lower-income households in accessing educational opportunities.

Disparities in educational opportunities contribute to a cycle of disadvantage that translates into health divides, leaving members of marginalized communities less equipped to invest in their health and navigate health crises. Even among those who are highly educated, good health is not guaranteed. Among college and graduate-level educated individuals, those from marginalized racial and ethnic groups still experience worse health, higher rates of chronic health conditions, higher infant and maternal mortality, and lower life expectancy compared to their white counterparts with similar levels of education.[23] In fact, a college-educated Black mother in the US has a higher chance of her infant dying than a white mother with less than a high school education.[24] Additional studies have shown that among highly educated individuals, those living in neighborhoods with high poverty, crime, and limited employment opportunities experience higher rates of cardiovascular disease, obesity, and mental health issues than those in more affluent areas.[25]

Why is this the case? While education can improve access to resources and increase health literacy, it does not ensure equal access to affordable, quality health care. Broader structural factors play a significant role, such as disparities in access to safe and affordable housing, green spaces, healthy food, and clean water; environmental pollution disproportionately concentrated in marginalized communities; and unequal systems and policies across education, housing, employment, and health care sectors. Furthermore, historical and systemic injustices such as residential segregation, Jim Crow laws, slavery, and colonialism have left impacts on health that persist regardless of the diplomas we earn.[26]

Most concerning, data show that disparities in mortality rates and life expectancy by education level have *widened* over the past several decades.[27] Even before the onset of COVID-19, the life expectancy gaps between US adults with the highest and lowest levels of education were at record highs.[28] By age 25, women with a graduate or professional degree were expected to live an additional 62 years, compared to just 50 years for women with less than a high school diploma—a staggering 12-year difference. For men, the education mortality gap is even more striking: those with advanced degrees were projected to live 60 more years, while their peers with less than a high school education were expected to live a whopping 16 fewer years. These stark contrasts reveal how strongly education is linked to life expectancy, and how these gaps have widened over time.

In the early weeks of the COVID-19 pandemic, government officials like New York's then governor Cuomo, celebrities, and others touted another "great equalizer"—that the virus affected all people equally and indiscriminately. This view, which soon proved false, drew on a long history of a "color-blind" approach to analyzing disasters that ignored or downplayed the role of systemic inequities in health. Socioeconomic disparities in infection and death rates have been well documented in prior pandemics, including the 1918, 1957, 1968, and 2009 influenza pandemics.[29] The people hit hardest were those in lower-paying jobs, such as essential workers, along with those living in densely populated urban areas with inadequate access to health care and public health resources. People like Marielis and her family. With history as a guide, public health experts warned that COVID-19 would exacerbate deep-seated income, occupational, and wealth inequities that would soon show up as health inequities.[30]

As COVID-19 exploded in New York City, Marielis never got used to the dread that gripped her chest when the wail of ambulance sirens pierced the air every few minutes—a reminder that many of her neighbors and family members living in other parts of New York City were getting sick. Marielis and her family did their best to physically distance from others, but that was almost impossible with scores of other residents sharing one run-down elevator, narrow stairwells, and cramped hallways of their aging six-story building. Essential workers like her sister had no choice but to go to work to continue paying the bills. Whether in health care, grocery stores, or public transportation, they faced an increased risk of exposure. On Zoom, Marielis could see the wealth divides in neat squares across her laptop. Those from wealthier families had more resources to weather the economic storm with family members who could work remotely (or not at all) and spacious, beautifully decorated homes where they could isolate if infected. She was thankful for the option to blur one's background.

What Marielis couldn't see—but doctors, nurses, and hospital workers in COVID hot spots could—was that most COVID patients in the intensive care units were people from lower-income neighborhoods like Marielis's and my own childhood neighborhood in Boston. At the time, many struggled to understand what public health experts saw clearly: COVID was spreading rapidly through poorer communities where physical distancing and working remotely were luxuries few could afford.

The pandemic, rather than acting as an equalizer, amplified existing injustices. Public health crises like the HIV/AIDS epidemic, the opioid crisis, and environmental disasters such as hurricanes, wildfires, and heat waves especially hurt marginalized groups,* not because of underlying biological or behavioral differences, but largely because of systems and policies that unfairly disadvantage or advantage people based on factors they have no control over: the circumstances into which they are born. And because this was predictable, research shows, it is also preventable.

Marginalized groups are those who experience social, economic, environmental, or political disadvantages because of their race, gender, socioeconomic status, disability, geographic location, sexual orientation, or other factors.

We can improve the health of our entire society and prevent the next public health crisis from being so devastating by investing in upstream approaches, rather than relying largely on downstream approaches. The upstream-downstream metaphor, credited to medical sociologist Irving Zola, illustrates this concept.[31] In this parable, a protagonist stands by a turbulent river where individuals keep falling in and drowning. Urgently, the protagonist begins rescuing each person from the water, but the effort quickly becomes overwhelming and the sheer volume of individuals drowning is too great to manage. The immediate demand to save lives also prevents the protagonist from traveling upstream to figure out why people are falling in the river in the first place.

Our society largely focuses on traditional downstream approaches, which address immediate health needs through the health care system, trying to rescue those who have already fallen into the fast-moving river. In contrast, upstream approaches focus on preventive policies and programs that put in guardrails to stop people from falling in.[32] A growing body of scientific research demonstrates that upstream interventions—those that target the social and structural determinants of health, such as safer housing, better neighborhood conditions, and removing barriers to socioeconomic opportunity—can successfully reduce health disparities and improve overall health.[33]

A core component of upstream solutions are policies aimed at improving social and economic conditions. Raising the minimum wage, for example, has been shown to lift families out of poverty and improve health by increasing access to essential resources like nutritious food, health care, and stable housing.[34] Providing affordable health care through policies like Medicaid expansion helps low-income households receive preventive care and treatment for chronic conditions, reducing mortality, increasing coverage, and improving overall health.[35] High-quality early childhood education programs that support children's growth in learning, emotional development, and social skills help set them up for success later in life. Children from low-income families who took part in these programs performed better in school, secured more stable jobs, and enjoyed better health as adults compared to their peers outside those programs.[36] These proactive measures improve well-being as well as reduce the long-term costs of treating preventable diseases.

When the COVID-19 pandemic hit, countries such as Taiwan, Vietnam, Hong Kong, Singapore, and Japan drew on prior experience with disease outbreaks (SARS in 2003, H1N1 influenza in 2009, and MERS in 2015) to swiftly enact both upstream and downstream interventions.[37] Many of these countries had already invested in robust upstream social safety nets, such as universal health care, paid sick leave, and expanded unemployment benefits, and were better equipped to handle the health and economic impacts of COVID-19. These proactive measures, combined with economic policies like enhanced unemployment benefits, targeted wage subsidies, and cash transfers to those in need reduced strain on health care systems, prevented widespread economic hardship, and saved more lives.[38]

Downstream efforts, which respond to the immediate needs of individuals once a crisis has occurred, also played a critical role in managing the pandemic. Countries like Singapore, with strong organizational infrastructure linking government and health care, focused on immediate measures such as creating accessible and widespread testing programs, using digital technology for rapid contact, and ramping up health care systems.[39] Additionally, many Asian nations combined early social control measures like travel restrictions, self-isolation, social distancing, and mask mandates with social and economic policies designed to protect low-income, rural, and other vulnerable communities.[40] These efforts allowed them to outperform the US in containing COVID-19.[41]

That's not what was happening in Marielis's Brooklyn, or in cities and towns across the US. While Marielis and her neighbors were battling the virus, they were also contending with preexisting health disparities tied to long-term socioeconomic struggles. Structural determinants such as overcrowded housing, limited health care access, and economic instability exacerbate health risks during crises. In her closet-sized half-bedroom, Marielis would hear the wail of sirens and pray it would move swiftly past her building. By the time the government and media acknowledged that the virus was disproportionately affecting the most vulnerable, Marielis and her family were still waking up to the sounds of ambulance sirens and coughing in the hallways—grim signs that another neighbor was falling ill or dying.

CHAPTER 2

The Spaces in Between

"Can Olivia and I have a playdate soon?" pleaded Jade, the younger of my two daughters, then seven, on a windy Saturday in March. She has hair the color of espresso, inquisitive eyes that are large and dark like her grandfather's, and a caramel complexion that deepens brilliantly during the warmer months.

"Which Olivia?" I asked.

"The one who is white," she said matter-of-factly.

Her sister, Ivy, then nine, raised an eyebrow and chimed in. "How do you know? Did you ask her?" She has chestnut-colored hair with natural sun-kissed highlights, almond-shaped light brown eyes that sparkle with mischief, and a peachy complexion that burns more easily than her sister's. Both carry my determined jaw, inherited Luke's long lanky limbs, and have delicate wavy curls, the kind of hair I dreamed of having when I was a child.

"No . . . but her skin is light," Jade said. Though her tone remained confident, a hint of uncertainty flickered across her face.

"Well, then you don't know for sure," Ivy said. "Look at me—my skin is light, but I am multiracial. You have to ask people what their race is."

Jade shot back. "Well, back in the old days, they would send you to the white schools and me to the Black schools, even though we're sisters. They wouldn't ask."

Luke and I exchanged a glance over the dinner table. Which one of us was going to take this?

Both of our daughters made valid points that reflect the evolving understanding of racial and ethnic identity. They are part of the 33.8 million and growing population of self-identified multiracial individuals in the US, according to the 2020 US Census.[1] Being married to Luke, who is multiracial, means that our children are Chinese, Irish, Black, and Native American.* They often ask if they are more Chinese, or more white, or more Black. We encourage them to embrace all aspects of their heritage, reminding them that they are a blend of both of us and our ancestors.

I tried to explain: "When we admire a rainbow, it's hard to tell exactly where each color starts and ends, like where the red blends into orange, and orange into yellow. We don't count how much blue there is compared to purple. It's the way the different colors come together seamlessly that make the rainbow whole and beautiful, just as each person's unique blend of backgrounds and ancestors makes up who they are."

Our young daughters' contrasting perspectives on race illustrate how the understanding and perception of race continue to change over time, from a more rigid, limited, and externally imposed categorization to a more nuanced and self-defined concept. But before we unpack how and why racial disparities exist in health, we must first establish a clear understanding of race and ethnicity.

Before the twentieth century, people thought of racial and ethnic groups as fixed, biological categories. In the early-to-mid-twentieth century, anthropologists like Franz Boas helped shift the perspective from viewing racial and ethnic groups as biological categories to seeing them as socially constructed, with a focus on cultural differences.[2] The Civil Rights Movement and other movements also played a significant role in emphasizing the socially constructed nature of these concepts.[3] Now, we understand *race* to be a concept rooted in historical, cultural, and societal perceptions that group people on how they appear.[4]

---

*Throughout this book, I use the word *Indigenous* to refer broadly to people who are native to their land (e.g., Indigenous people in Australia, New Zealand, Hawaii, Alaska, Canada, Mexico). When I refer specifically to people Indigenous to the continental US I use *Native American*, which is what my relatives prefer to use. When drawing from different sources, however, I may choose to use the phrasing used by those sources, such as "American Indian."

One current definition of *race* is a group to which people belong (or are perceived to belong), based on certain shared physical characteristics, such as skin color, hair texture, and facial features.[5] *Ethnicity*, derived from the Greek word "ethnos" (meaning "nation"), refers to a group to which people belong (or are perceived to belong) as a result of shared cultural factors such as nationality, language, ancestry, religion, and traditions. Both are complex, multidimensional, and ever-changing concepts shaped by society, with layers of meaning and interpretation that shift depending on time and place.

The modern concept of "race" emerged during the colonial expansions of European nations between the sixteenth and eighteenth centuries, with its definition largely based on superficial characteristics such as skin color.[6] While human civilization has existed for millennia, it was during this historical period that global racial categorizations began to form, influencing Western-imposed perceptions, racial hierarchies, and discriminatory practices.[7] In different parts of the world, the twenty-first-century concept of race is measured and defined differently. For example, before 1985, Japan's policy for assigning race on a child's birth certificate was paternalistic, deferring to the race and nationality of the father to determine the race of the child.[8] In Brazil, mixed race has been recognized as early as its first census in 1872, where an estimated 38.3 percent of Brazilians that year identified as "Pardo" (of mixed or multiple ethnic ancestries).[9] Racial measurement in the Brazilian census focuses primarily on skin color,[10] with as many as twelve or more categories available for self-identification.[11]

In the US, the legacy of the "one-drop" rule, which evolved in the nineteenth century, persisted well into the 1980s, shaping both legal and social classifications of racial identity. Rooted in the history of slavery and Jim Crow laws, the one-drop rule dictated that anyone with even a single Black ancestor was considered Black, irrespective of their appearance or other ancestral backgrounds.[12] Many states codified this rule into law to prevent light-skinned multiracial individuals from passing as white. For example, Arkansas passed Act 320 (House Bill 79) in 1911, which defined as "Negro" anyone "who has . . . any negro blood whatever."[13] Such rigid, anti-Black categorizations were used to enforce racial segregation and discrimination in housing, employment, education, health care, voting rights, criminal justice, and other areas of daily life.

Enforcement of the one-drop rule is a form of *structural racism*—systems, policies, and practices that perpetuate racial inequality and disadvantage certain racial groups—with pervasive and often harsh effects. The one-drop rule was used to justify discriminatory practices such as denying people of color and multiracial individuals access to education, housing, employment opportunities, and public facilities reserved for white people.[14] Laws and social customs based on this rule upheld unfair social hierarchies based on skin color. The one-drop rule also served to maintain the "purity" of whiteness by ensuring that anyone with even a trace of Black ancestry was excluded from the privileges and benefits associated with whiteness.

The very definition and organization of "race" itself is a form of structural discrimination, profoundly shaping the experiences of individuals and communities while perpetuating racial disparities in education, employment, housing, health care, and other domains throughout history. This structural bias is evident in past and current restrictions on racial self-identification on official forms, like the inability to check off more than one race on the US Census before 2000. For my husband and our daughters, this meant facing pressure to fit into narrow racial classifications that fail to capture their full identities and ancestry. As my husband grew up in the '90s and early aughts, teachers and nurses frequently urged him to simply check the box for Black on standardized tests and health forms, disregarding his multiracial background.

Even in 2021, as I hurried online to sign up for a COVID-19 vaccine for myself, Luke, and our girls as soon as it became available, the race and ethnicity question popped up on my phone from the online pharmacy portal. Check one:

☐ White
☐ Hispanic/Latino/a
☐ Asian
☐ Black
☐ Native American/American Indian
☐ Other

On a personal level, it seemed straightforward to select "Asian" for myself, but on a professional level, I knew that grouping all Asians and Pacific

Islanders into one monolith hides important socioeconomic, behavioral, and health differences between subgroups like Chinese, Vietnamese, Filipino, and Asian Indian. For example, a review disaggregating twenty-four Asian American subgroups found significant disparities in cancer, heart disease, mental health, and more across these groups.[15] These distinctions, however, are often masked when people are lumped together under the broad label of Asian American Pacific Islander.

I also hesitated over which race to select on the vaccine registration form for Luke and our daughters. I didn't know how this data would be used. How could a policymaker, researcher, or clinician make sense of data from people forced to check off a category as nondescript as "Other"? My family, like millions of others across the world, belongs in multiple categories and in the spaces in between. Even when given the option to self-identify in a more nuanced and comprehensive way, it doesn't always align with how others perceive and treat us.

This issue persists in many settings, including the doctor's office, a place where patients seek compassion, humanity, and respect. A few years ago, Luke took Ivy to see a new pediatrician for a routine checkup. When they returned, she showed no signs that anything was amiss, but he was visibly unsettled. While she played with her toys upstairs, I asked him how the visit went.

"You should have seen how the nurse and pediatrician changed their attitudes towards me once I explained I was a doctor. They wouldn't even look me in the eye when we first came in."

Though I wasn't there, I could imagine the scenario unfolding—the shift from disengagement to surprise, then warmth, followed by full engagement. Standing an entire foot taller than me with an athletic build, Luke has hazel eyes that reflect green or amber depending on what he wears and tan skin that deepens effortlessly under the sun—a seamless blend of his parents. He is tall, dark, and handsome on any day (and I say this as a scientist, so I can claim no bias). On that particular day, he was wearing a casual hoodie and sweatpants.

Whether in person, online, or on paper, how we are treated is profoundly shaped by how others perceive our racial and ethnic identity. Research shows, for example, that people often make assumptions about others' social class based on their perceived race,[16] leading to disparities in how individuals are treated and the opportunities and barriers presented to them. Using race as a proxy for socioeconomic status, for instance, by assuming that a Black person has lower levels of education and income, or perhaps is more likely to be a "difficult" patient, is highly problematic for a few reasons. One, while race and socioeconomic status are intertwined due to structural racism, they are not interchangeable. Simply put, belonging to a particular racial group doesn't dictate one's socioeconomic status, and vice versa. Second, it overlooks the complex realities of people's lives, including the socioeconomic hardships that people across all racial and ethnic groups may face. Third and most importantly, it perpetuates harmful assumptions, stereotypes, and actions, as well as undermines efforts to recognize and address the root causes of racial disparities in health.

Research consistently highlights the strong connection between race, ethnicity, and health. While socioeconomic status is a major contributor to health, it doesn't fully account for the racial disparities observed. For instance, studies show that college-educated Black and Hispanic/Latino people suffer from higher rates of chronic health conditions, higher premature all-cause mortality, and lower life expectancy than their similarly educated white counterparts.[17] Even when controlling for factors like income, education, and health care access, racial disparities in health persist across numerous outcomes—from infant mortality to life expectancy, from chronic diseases like cancer to infectious diseases like COVID.[18] Decades of data challenge the belief that socioeconomic status alone can explain the health inequities experienced across racial lines. This research has prompted many to explore other factors that drive racial disparities, including genetics and biology.

For centuries, physicians, researchers, and the public have debated the extent to which genetic or biological differences among "racial" groups explain the health disparities we observe, especially given that white populations, on the whole, tend to live healthier, longer lives than people of color. One example of this is the enduring belief that people of African descent are "naturally" more prone to developing high blood pressure. This notion, however, has been challenged by substantial research from fields spanning genetics, epidemiology, and medicine. One compelling research strategy is to compare the health of people from similar and different racial groups across different countries. This allows us to see whether racial disparities in health remain consistent or vary depending on where people live.

Extensive analyses produced surprising results. A 2005 study surveyed 85,000 European- and African-descent adults across ten countries: US, Canada, Italy, Sweden, Germany, England, Finland, Spain, Nigeria, and Jamaica.[19] The rates of hypertension among individuals of European-descent (27–55 percent) and African-descent (14–44 percent) varied only modestly between racial groups. While hypertension rates were higher among Black individuals in the US, they were lower among Black populations in Jamaica and Nigeria. This multinational study was among the first to suggest that factors beyond genetic ancestry, such as social and environmental determinants of health, may play a more significant role in determining health than "race" alone.

In 2004, *Nature* published a groundbreaking series of studies investigating genetic variation across human populations and its implications for health.[20] One study analyzed the genetic diversity within and between populations and found that the variation within so-called major "racial" groups was often greater than the variation between them, suggesting that genetic differences between "races" are minimal. Another study examined the genetic basis of common diseases like diabetes, heart disease, and cancer, finding that genetic risk factors were distributed across populations without clear racial patterns. This indicates that genetic predispositions to these conditions are shaped by a complex interplay of environmental, lifestyle, and genetic factors. The research also highlighted that social determinants, such as socioeconomic status and health care access, have a far greater impact on population health and health disparities than genetic differences between racial groups.

This collection of research challenges the idea that "inherent" genetic differences across racial groups are the primary cause of racial health disparities, emphasizing instead the role of social and structural determinants of health such as racism and the ways it manifests. Dr. Camara Jones, a leading public health researcher, physician, and epidemiologist known globally for her work on racism and health disparities, developed a framework outlining three levels of racism: internalized, personally mediated, and institutionalized.[21] This framework helps us understand how racism operates at different levels of society and affects individuals and communities in distinct ways. Of the two, personally mediated and internalized racism are perhaps the most readily visible in everyday life. I will focus on those two levels in the remainder of this chapter and turn to institutional racism in the next.

My mother-in-law, Reese, is tough as nails yet never without a sense of poise. She is tall with vivid blue eyes, has fair skin that freckles in the summer, and has shoulder-length buttery-blond hair. There is a sharpness in her gaze, an unspoken confidence that makes it clear she doesn't back down. The oldest of six daughters in a working-class Irish American family, she was born in 1954 (the same year that Ruby Bridges was born) and grew up in Worcester, Massachusetts, the second-largest city in the state.

My father-in-law, Mitch, had a towering figure with dark skin the color of cocoa, large expressive eyes that seemed to take in everything, and rough hands shaped by years of carpentry work. In the 1970s, he grew an Afro and a beard that only added to his striking presence. Tall and trim were just about the only traits Reese and Mitch shared. With her outgoing nature and charisma, Reese could strike up a conversation with anyone she met. Mitch was quiet and stoic, his hearty laughs and goofy humor typically reserved for close family, friends, and bowling buddies. He had started supporting his family (a blend of African American and Native American ancestry) at the age of ten when his own father passed.

They married in 1980, just thirteen years after the historic *Loving v. Virginia* ruling that legalized interracial marriage in the US. They stood out as one of the few interracial marriages in their community. Together, they navigated a world that often struggled to accept their union.

"We stayed in Worcester where there were other families of color," Reese recounted. "That's why I never moved to the suburbs. We didn't go to certain restaurants or clubs where we knew we wouldn't be welcome. And I always made sure to go to the hospital with him. Each time, I'd go right up to the staff and immediately say, 'I'm his wife, here is our insurance.'"

In 2014, this turned out to not be enough. Mitch had been having severe abdominal pain and noticed blood in his stool. When he voiced his concerns, his primary care physician told him it was likely hemorrhoids. Both Reese and Luke, with the latter in his last year of medical school, convinced Mitch to go to the emergency room to get his pain checked out. The first doctor they saw was a white man in his sixties.

"He thought Mitch was an alcoholic when we described his pain, though I explained to him that this was not the case," Reese recalled. "He sent us home with pills for indigestion. No tests, no referrals. Mitch didn't want to make a fuss and hated hospitals, so we left." The doctor also failed to recognize that Mitch was overdue for colon cancer screening and overlooked both the severity of his pain and the fact that he had been experiencing bloody stools for months.

A few months later, they rushed back. The pills did nothing, the pain had not subsided, and Mitch had begun throwing up his bowel movements.

Reese said, "This time I went up to the staff and I said, 'I'm his wife, here is our insurance, and our son is in medical school here.' You should have seen them move."

That day, they saw a different doctor, who promptly ordered a CT scan. The tests came back, revealing a devastating diagnosis: stage 4 colon cancer. Mitch had been suffering from pain for nearly a year. A CT scan could have been ordered much earlier, raising painful questions about how many warning signs went unnoticed. Over the next four years, he went through the best cancer treatment available, with Reese by his side every step of the way. In 2018, the cancer spread, he developed an infection, and one of his lungs collapsed. In his final weeks, though he could barely speak or move, he still summoned the strength to stand and greet his youngest granddaughter, Jade, who had recently turned one.

"She reminds me of my mom. I wish they could have met," he said softly, his voice filled with a pride and sadness.

———

My in-laws were all too familiar with *personally mediated racism*. Reese saw it whenever she was with Mitch, and he experienced it throughout his life. This level of racism refers to discriminatory actions, behaviors, or attitudes exhibited by individuals toward others based on their perceived race or ethnicity. In health care, this can manifest in health care professionals treating patients differently because of their race, as was the case with my late father-in-law. It can look like spending less time with patients, asking fewer questions, dismissing or undervaluing their concerns, deciding further testing or specialty referrals are not needed, refusing care, or making assumptions about patients' intentions and behaviors that influence quality of care and decision-making.

The health impacts of racial discrimination from people in health care and other settings are profound. A landmark 2007 study published the results of a blinded study where 287 physicians were randomized to view a clinical scenario about a patient who arrives at the emergency room with severe heart concerns.[22] The physicians were given identical patient scenarios, histories, and profiles, with the only difference being the patient's race (either white or Black). The findings revealed that physicians showed bias in favor of white patients and held stereotypes of Black patients as less cooperative. Alarmingly, physicians with stronger pro-white bias were more likely to treat white patients and neglect to treat Black patients.

Beyond that scenario-based study, the implicit racial bias and unequal treatment in health care are also reflected in real life. A systematic review of health care professionals found that most exhibit positive attitudes toward white patients and negative attitudes toward Black, Hispanic/ Latino, and darker-skinned patients, and this bias significantly impacted patient-provider interactions, treatment decisions, treatment adherence, and patient health.[23] For example, clinicians' belief that white patients are more likely to follow treatment plans led to delayed prescriptions for patients of color compared to their white peers. Numerous studies have documented health care professionals' dismissing pain symptoms in people of color, particularly women of color.[24] The disparate care that patients of color receive can lead to delayed diagnoses, higher rates of misdiagnoses, inadequate treatment, and ultimately worse health.

This unequal treatment creates a vicious cycle. Experiencing discrimination is linked to delaying or avoiding seeking health care like my father-in-law, and also to postponing preventive services like cholesterol testing, blood tests and eye exams to monitor diabetes, and flu shots.[25] Research including my own also show that people who experience discrimination based on race, ethnicity, gender, or other factors often experience increased levels of stress, anxiety, depression, and other mental health issues.[26] This chronic stress can lead to physiological changes in the body, such as high blood pressure, inflammation, elevated cortisol levels, and weakened immune function, all of which increase the risk of chronic conditions such as cardiovascular disease and diabetes.[27] Experiencing discrimination can also lead to unhealthy coping behaviors such as substance use, poor dietary habits, and decreased physical activity.[28]

In the early 2010s, scientists made groundbreaking discoveries that revealed how experiencing discrimination can affect our bodies, down to the level of our DNA. This discovery supported Dr. Arline Geronimus's earlier weathering hypothesis, suggesting that the constant stress from discrimination, poverty, exposure to violence, and other life adversities can cause wear and tear on the body in a phenomenon called allostatic load.[29] Recent studies found that racism is linked with shorter telomeres, adding to research showing that chronic stress from racism is associated with higher allostatic load.[30] Telomeres, which are the protective caps on the ends of our chromosomes (like shoelace caps), help keep our cells healthy and stable as they divide over time. Study participants who experience chronic stress from discrimination showed accelerated telomere shortening.[31] This can speed up biological aging and increase vulnerability to chronic diseases like cancer and heart disease. While most of the research has focused on adults, I also wondered about the impact of these stressors on children.

"Hey, Mommy?" asked Jade one night a few years ago. She was four, and bedtime question-time remains a favorite routine of ours. During this time, she and her sister could talk about anything they wanted.

"Yes?" I said.

"I want to have white skin like you and Ivy, not brown like Daddy's."

Her words felt like a gut punch, knocking the wind out of me. For a heartbeat, I was silent. I knew my children would internalize centuries-old societal attitudes around lighter versus darker skin tones, but hearing it so directly hit me hard. It wasn't lost on me that her lighter-skinned sister had never expressed a desire for darker skin.

I reassured her. "Your skin is beautiful. It's one of the parts about you I love most. It reminds me of warm sunshine and cinnamon. I love how you get extra toasty in the summer."

"Mmmmmm . . . thanks, Mommy. You're the best," murmured Jade sleepily before drifting off.

I shut the door gently, made my way downstairs, and silently wept, knowing that this would be the first of many conversations she and I would have on something she has no control over—how she is seen by the outside world.

―――――――

Internalized racism is the acceptance of negative stereotypes and beliefs about one's own racial or ethnic group as true. Studies show that as early as children can speak, they begin to internalize the belief that those with lighter-skinned are better and more deserving than those with darker skin.[32] This form of racism influences how people see themselves, impacting how they function and their mental and physical health. A randomized trial in the US demonstrated that when college students were told they belonged to a group expected to perform poorly on exams, their exam scores suffered.[33] For example, Black students who were told that Black students typically perform worse on a specific exam than white students, women who were told they perform worse than men, and white students who were told they usually do worse than Asian students, all scored lower on tests compared to groups who were not exposed to such messages.[34] Beyond academic performance, the stigma of racial inferiority and internalized racism is linked with higher blood pressure and psychological distress among Black participants.[35]

In health care, internalized racism can result in individuals from marginalized communities to believe that they are inherently less deserving of quality care, or that certain health issues like heart disease and diabetes are inevitable for their racial group. This internalization may lead a person of color to avoid seeking medical help or withhold concerns from health care professionals, as Mitch often did.

From deeply internalized beliefs to the interpersonal marginalization people face, all the way up to the institutionalized systems that govern our lives (systems we'll explore in the next chapter) these interconnected levels of racism profoundly shape how we are born, live, and die. As a parent, I see the beauty and potential equally in my children, yet I'm painfully aware that they will encounter unequal treatment based on their appearance. As a public health expert, I know there are evidence-based practices and interventions we can put into action, along with new strategies to explore. For this chapter, we will focus on interventions delivered at the interpersonal and individual levels.

One powerful approach for communities of color involves *empowerment-based interventions*, which equip individuals or communities with the tools and knowledge they need to take charge of their lives, make informed choices, and actively improve their well-being.[36] This approach can be especially helpful for low-income communities of color, as it builds confidence, independence, and the ability to create positive changes, even when resources are limited.[37] Tailored to specific cultural contexts, these methods acknowledge systemic injustices, encourage participant involvement in decision-making, and strengthen community connection. Research shows that empowerment-based interventions can help improve the health of communities of color, with benefits seen in depressive symptoms,[38] diet and physical activity,[39] safe sex practices,[40] and body mass index.[41] At the individual level, practicing self-affirmation techniques, like positive self-talk, has been shown to help individuals better cope with stress and make healthier choices.[42]

Another set of interventions includes *implicit bias trainings*, which aim to raise awareness of unconscious biases and offer strategies to address them, and culturally competent trainings that seek to improve understanding of cultural backgrounds and provide effective communication. Yet, the effectiveness of these trainings varies.[43] Some studies show reduced biased behavior among health care providers, educators, and other professionals,[44] while research shows little or no improvement.[45] One reason for these mixed results could be the variation in how these programs are structured. These inconsistencies could stem from differences in the topics covered, objectives, delivery methods, and evaluation practices.

My colleagues and I conducted a yearlong systematic review to assess the effectiveness of diversity, equity, inclusion, and antiracism training interventions across various work settings, including health care.[46] Our objective was to analyze the scope, methodologies, and outcomes of these interventions to better understand their impact and identify factors that contribute to their success or limitations. Our review revealed that most studies involved a single training session, with significant variability in content, goals, assessment methods, and effectiveness.

We discussed several approaches to enhance the impact of these trainings in the workplace. These included prioritizing long-term learning over onetime sessions, standardizing assessment methods, and ensuring consistent evaluations of efforts. Rather than focusing only on surface-level knowledge and attitudes, trainings can emphasize the development of critical skills relevant for all professionals. Key skills include culturally competent communication (promoting an understanding of and respect for a variety of cultural backgrounds), conflict resolution (navigating differing viewpoints to foster collaborative solutions), stereotype discrediting (challenging oversimplified beliefs with accurate information), emotional intelligence (improving relationships through better understanding and management of emotions), and perspective taking (enhancing empathy by considering others' viewpoints and experiences).

Additionally, these programs could involve communities in the design, delivery, and evaluation of these programs, while fostering advocacy, community organizing, and policy change. This, in turn, can lead to more relevant and sustainable solutions, strengthening community resilience in the long term.[47]

While these interventions may offer some relief, they are ultimately a temporary fix, a Band-Aid to stop the bleed of a deep wound. Beyond individual and interpersonal efforts, we must swim even further upstream to tackle institutionalized, structural, and systemic racism—the kinds that can be harder to see (and therefore dismantle) because they are all around us. Take another breath, and let's dive in.

CHAPTER 3

A Tale of
Two Neighborhoods

On a sweltering August afternoon in 1993, I found myself sitting in a small, ground floor office in an old building, my eight-year-old body restless in a stiff, itchy polyester dress. Heat, humidity, and I never got along. My only solace was the faintest whisper of a warm breeze through the open window. Across from me sat a Black woman, her warm smile and stylish buzzed '90s haircut instantly putting me at ease. She was interviewing me for the Metropolitan Council for Educational Opportunity (METCO) program, the longest-running voluntary school desegregation (busing) program in the US.

Born from a commitment to improve educational opportunity in the wake of school segregation, METCO primarily serves students of color, offering them the ability to attend schools in more affluent suburban districts. Acceptance is based on a mix of factors: space availability, the student's academic record, and priority for students who meet certain criteria such as socioeconomic status or educational need. This initiative was more than just a bus ride to a different school—it represented a path to go beyond the limitations of inner-city zip codes. It offered students like me the chance to attend well-resourced public schools in suburban districts—schools that boasted smaller class sizes, up-to-date textbooks, advanced coursework, extracurricular activities, and a wealth of opportunities that were often unavailable in our underfunded Boston public schools.

Unable to afford private school tuition or relocate to a neighborhood with better schools, my dad sought out alternatives and came across

METCO. As I sat in that cramped office, the interview questions flowed one right after the other. She wanted to know about me—my hobbies, my favorite books, the school subjects that sparked my curiosity. I felt like I was being tested but didn't know if I gave the correct answers.

A few weeks later, the news came: I had been accepted into the METCO program and would be attending a new school in the fall, one that was ten miles away and would require a round-trip three-hour school bus ride. That moment marked the beginning of a journey that would shape my future in ways I couldn't yet understand.

As I was a second-grade student about to enter third, the complexities of METCO eluded me. I didn't understand why most of my METCO peers were Black or Hispanic/Latino, or the history behind the program. I also didn't realize I would be one of the few Asian students until I stepped onto the school bus for the first time. What I did understand was my parents' unwavering determination for me to receive the best education possible.

From third to twelfth grade, my life as a METCO student was a tale of two worlds. My family and I lived in a modest, rent-controlled townhouse next to the projects in Roslindale, a mixed-income, ethnically diverse neighborhood in Boston. Meanwhile, my school was in Belmont, a picturesque, affluent suburb known for its top-tier public schools. The daily commute was long. It meant school bus rides in elementary school, then public transit once middle school hit. I woke up before 6 a.m. to catch the bus and returned home just before dinner.

"It's worth the sacrifice," my dad would say whenever I complained about the commute and the challenges of navigating two vastly different environments. Education, he insisted, offered the pathway to stability and prestige—advantages my parents were born without. Yet, confronted with the stark contrasts of privilege and disadvantage daily, I found myself wondering: How can education alone bridge such a gap when the inequality between these worlds felt so deep?

The two neighborhoods I commuted between, just ten miles apart, might as well have been worlds apart. In Boston, my METCO peers and I understood the unspoken rules: avoid the parks after dusk, steer clear of certain streets. We saw theft and assault, and we were often verbally and physically harassed on our school commutes. The streets were lined with the garish colors of fast-food joints, liquor stores, and corner shops; the sidewalks were cracked, and the air near Washington Street, where we waited for the bus to Forest Hills station, was thick with vehicle exhaust.

Belmont, on the other hand, painted a picture of idyllic suburban life. Many of my majority-white classmates walked or rode bikes to school on smooth, safe, tree-lined streets; carried colorful lunches packed with fruits and vegetables to school; spent afternoons in expensive arts and athletics programs; and, for some, received brand-new cars for their sixteenth birthdays.

I spent the least amount of time with the kids who lived in my neighborhood and attended schools in Boston. These children shared similar economic backgrounds to my own family and were racially and ethnically diverse. There were the Irish American twins next door, the Venezuelan American family across the street, and the Haitian American family a few doors down, all raised by single mothers. Of all the neighborhood kids in our rent-controlled community, I was closest with Maria, a teenager with glorious mahogany curls, a lilting accent, and a smile that radiated warmth and kindness. She was fiercely protective of her older brother, Javi, who was cognitively impaired and often the target of teasing. Maria's house became the first refuge I sought when one day, while taking public transit home from middle school, I was harassed and followed by older teenagers.

"What's your name? You're pretty. Come on, why won't you talk with us?"

I was twelve years old in the late '90s (cell phones were rare), unsettled and terrified at the two older boys who wouldn't leave me alone at the Forest Hills station. They boarded the bus with me and stared the entire ride, their eyes unsmiling and their mouths twisted in smirks. Their casual disregard for my discomfort turned my stomach into knots. When my stop finally came, I got off the bus, but to my horror, one of the boys followed me. Trying not to panic, I rushed to Maria's house instead of mine, hoping her family would be there. Luckily, her mom was home. She let me wait inside until the harasser gave up and left. Despite her limited English, she sensed my distress, brushed away my tears, and walked me home. I couldn't sleep well for days and dreaded running into the boys again on public transit.

Three sets of children, families, and communities in varying contexts; three distinct social, racial, economic, environmental, and health realities.

Not only was the community in Belmont whiter and wealthier than my METCO peers—they seemed healthier too. Far fewer of them struggled with chronic conditions like asthma or diabetes, conditions that affected several of my METCO peers and neighbors in Boston. As we entered adolescence, struggles with weight gain and mental health took a higher toll on commuting students of color. Those living in my neighborhood attending Boston's public schools faced even greater challenges, including lower educational attainment, limited job prospects, higher rates of tobacco and substance use, and poorer overall health.

It wasn't until adulthood that I learned stories like mine could be found in every city across the nation. From the East Coast to the West, children of different socioeconomic and racial backgrounds are growing up worlds apart—sometimes just miles from each other. A groundbreaking study, the Child Opportunity Index 3.0, shines a light on this divide. By examining data from over 73,000 census tracts nationwide, it highlights disparities in three key areas: education, health and environment, and social and economic factors, assigning each neighborhood a Child Opportunity Score from 1 to 100.[1]

The findings are eye opening: In the 100 largest metro areas, disparities in opportunity are glaring. While white children in the US typically live in neighborhoods with a respectable opportunity score of 74, Black and Hispanic/Latino children often live in areas with scores as low as 30 or 33, respectively. This index, unveiled in 2024 by the diversitydatakids.org initiative at Brandeis University, spotlights the widespread neighborhood inequities by race. How did this come to be? Were communities of color always less desirable than white communities? Why were programs like METCO created for students of color?

To answer these questions, let's take a brief trip through US housing history. During the economic turmoil of the Great Depression, banks were reluctant to provide housing loans, leaving many families struggling to buy homes and 2 million construction workers without jobs. In response, President Franklin Roosevelt established the Home Owners' Loan Corporation (HOLC) in 1933 and the Federal Housing Administration (FHA) in 1934 as part of the New Deal to stabilize the economy, create new jobs, and provide financial assistance to homeowners.[2] The HOLC was made to stabilize the housing market by focusing primarily on refinancing home mortgages that were in default or at risk of foreclosure. The FHA was created to stimulate the housing market by providing mortgage insurance to lenders, making it easier for homebuyers to qualify for loans and for lenders to extend credit. This helped increase homeownership rates by reducing the risk for lenders and providing more favorable terms for borrowers.

Over the next several years, HOLC surveyors went to neighborhoods across the country, looking for signs of neglect and decay and noting if the residents included Black people, Jewish people, or immigrants from Italy, Ireland, and other European countries. Using these evaluations, the HOLC created thousands of secret residential maps that color-coded neighborhoods by grades of "residential security."[3] Colors signaled the perceived riskiness of lending in those areas.[4] Areas that were coded green were the first grade; these areas were noted to be free of Black and "foreign-born white" residents, and lenders were encouraged to offer the maximum loan amount for properties. Blue was the second grade; lenders were advised to make loans 10–15 percent below the maximum in these areas. The third grade was yellow; these areas were considered at risk of "infiltration of a lower-grade population." And the fourth grade was marked in red, indicating areas where lenders frequently refused to offer loans—areas that were often predominantly Black. These redlined neighborhoods were often located near downtown, next to factories, railroad tracks, and bus terminals.

It is widely believed that the FHA played a key role in reinforcing these discriminatory practices by adopting the HOLC's color-coded maps and using them to determine which neighborhoods were eligible for mortgage insurance.[5] Yet, more recent analyses suggest that the FHA began discriminating against low-income urban neighborhoods (which were predominantly Black) even before the HOLC created these maps.[6] Regardless of the timeline, low-income communities of color were often excluded from FHA-backed mortgages.

It wasn't until I was twenty-two, in public health graduate school at Harvard, that I first learned about redlining as a form of *institutionalized racism*. This term refers to discriminatory practices and policies embedded within institutions like government agencies, banks, real estate, and the judicial system that systematically disadvantage specific racial or ethnic groups.[7] Redlining led to the creation and perpetuation of racially segregated neighborhoods, devaluing properties in neighborhoods with predominantly Black, Hispanic/Latino, and immigrant residents while artificially inflating property values in predominantly white neighborhoods. Redlining is also an example of structural racism, as discussed in the prior chapter.[8]

Structural racism in housing and home ownership has had far-reaching consequences. In areas marked as high risk, residents faced obstacles in obtaining mortgage loans or insurance, or were charged higher interest rates. Consequently, many families of color, particularly Black families, were excluded from homeownership opportunities and the ability to build wealth,[9] key indicators of socioeconomic status linked to health, as discussed in chapter 2. Nearly a hundred years later, Black American families in 2023 still have the lowest rates of homeownership (45.9 percent) compared to non-Hispanic/Latino white Americans (73.8 percent), Asian Americans (63 percent), and Hispanic/Latino Americans (49.8 percent).[10] In 2022, the average wealth of white families soared to $1.4 million, while Black families trailed significantly behind at about $211,000 and Hispanic/Latino families at $227,000.[11] This $1 million gap is the widest to date, illustrating the persistent wealth divide by racial groups.

In redlined areas, the devaluation of properties created a cycle of economic decline. One significant impact was the decline in property tax revenue, as properties in redlined neighborhoods were often assessed at lower values compared to those in green or blue areas. With lower property tax revenue, local governments had fewer resources to invest in essential public services, such as education. As a result, public school systems in redlined areas often faced chronic underfunding and resource shortages.[12] This lack of investment translated into poorer educational opportunities for students, including outdated facilities, less competitive salaries to attract and retain high-quality teachers, limited access to educational materials, and fewer extracurricular activities.[13] A 2020 report found that school districts primarily serving white students received $23 *billion* more in funding than those serving predominantly students of color in the US.[14] Consequently, in redlined neighborhoods in Boston and across the country, public school students face substantial educational disadvantage compared to their peers in wealthier, predominantly white areas. These educational disadvantages result from cycles of socioeconomic disadvantages that were artificially and unfairly mapped onto racial lines.

With limited access to loans and financial resources, redlined communities struggled to invest in essential infrastructure such as roads, public transportation, parks, utilities, and community facilities.[15] At the same time, the negative stigma associated with these neighborhoods discouraged investors and businesses from establishing themselves there. This included essential goods and services like grocery stores and pharmacies. Businesses offering fresh produce, fitness facilities, and health care were more likely to establish themselves in "desirable" neighborhoods, assuming residents there would have more disposable income to spend on such services. This trend further entrenched neighborhood disparities by limiting access to key factors that promote health, such as safe green spaces, essential services, and access to affordable fresh produce. Over time, this led to stark differences in the living conditions and available services in neighborhoods that can be traced back to the HOLC's color-coded maps.

Physical environment and neighborhood health. Our health is profoundly impacted by our physical environment, such as the quality of the air we breathe, the water we drink, the walkability of our neighborhoods, and the green spaces we can access. Decades of research show that structural racism in housing has driven deterioration of the physical environment in redlined communities. These neighborhoods suffer from higher levels of pollution, substandard housing, and environmental hazards like limited green spaces, fewer trees, increased airborne hazards,[16] and higher temperatures.[17] These unhealthy conditions can then lead to more asthma-related emergency room visits and chronic respiratory problems, as well as other health issues linked to poor environmental surroundings.[18]

Service environment and neighborhood health. Our neighborhood environments are also characterized by the services they provide or lack. Redlined neighborhoods often lack essential services and resources that support good health. These communities are often designated as food deserts and have few, if any, grocery stores[19] and recreational fitness resources, with higher density of fast-food and alcohol outlets.[20] Living in such environments makes it far more challenging to maintain healthy behaviors, increasing risk for chronic conditions like hypertension, diabetes, and heart disease. The lack of health care services and adequate infrastructure further compounds these risks. A systematic review and meta-analysis found that redlined areas experience worse health outcomes, including higher rates of pre-term births and multiple chronic conditions.[21]

Social environment and neighborhood health. A neighborhood's social environment, such as the presence of violence, chronic stressors, and the availability of social support networks, also shapes our health. High levels of violence and chronic stress, and a lack of support systems, negatively affects mental and physical health.[22] Historical disinvestment, economic hardship, and systemic inequality in redlined neighborhoods contribute to higher rates of violence and stress in these areas.[23] Limits to resources such as job opportunities, quality schools, and safe public spaces fuel instability that raises stress levels and can drive up violence and crime.[24] Additionally, residents may experience social isolation due to economic strain and inadequate social services, which erodes community trust and cohesion.[25]

Over time, the unhealthy physical, service, and social environments along with other structural inequities created by racial residential segregation has led to higher rates of hypertension, diabetes, obesity, cardiovascular disease, chronic respiratory diseases, compromised immune systems, cancer, and premature death that persists today.[26]

As the COVID-19 pandemic unfolded, it magnified the health disparities stemming from structural racism. A study in New York City revealed that historically redlined neighborhoods, like the one Marielis lived in, experienced significantly higher rates of COVID-19 infection than non-redlined areas.[27] Additional research confirmed that redlined neighborhoods have higher rates of preexisting conditions that increase COVID-19 complications, such as asthma, chronic obstructive pulmonary disease, diabetes, and obesity.[28] These disparities are linked to social determinants of health heavily influenced by the legacy of redlining, such as overcrowded housing and limited access to health care, pharmacies, and healthy food.[29] While redlining was officially outlawed in 1968 with the passage of the Fair Housing Act, its legacy continues to deeply impact the health of residents across generations.

In recent years, redlining has manifested in more modern forms, especially digital redlining. *Digital redlining* is a discriminatory practice by internet service providers and technology companies that involves restricting access to, or increasing the cost of, high-speed internet and digital resources in neighborhoods due to socioeconomic or demographic factors. Just as redlining in housing denied communities of color essential resources and opportunities, digital redlining denies access to the digital infrastructure necessary for information, education, employment, health care, and civic engagement. Data from Los Angeles County revealed that race and income were directly linked to where internet service providers chose to invest in broadband, with less competition for service in low-income and Black neighborhoods.[30] In 2023, more than 42 million people in the nation did not have high-speed internet, and redlined, rural, and low-income communities bore the heaviest burden of this digital divide.

Digital redlining is an invisible structural determinant of health that worsens health and health inequities.[31] Redlined communities face greater barriers to accessing online health services due to limited internet and device availability, exacerbating racial and neighborhood disparities in preventive care and managing chronic diseases. During the distribution of COVID-19 vaccines, online registration excluded people without reliable internet and digital devices, hitting low-income communities of color harder. Digital disparities also limit access to health information, delay communication with health care providers, and impede remote monitoring of health conditions.

The tragic irony in the prevailing legacy of redlining lies in the fact that, before 1933, the belief that communities of color lived in less desirable neighborhoods was largely unfounded. This perception, however, was manufactured into reality after the federal government, banking, real estate, insurance, and other business sectors embraced the HOLC's color-coded maps. The story of redlining vividly illustrates how structural racism in housing significantly shapes racial health disparities.

If racism existed within only housing, we would not see the extent of racial inequities in health that persist today. Instead, the scale of disparities is driven by the widespread and ongoing interconnection of structural racism across multiple domains, including education, employment, the legal system, health care, and voting rights. This is what is known as *systemic racism*—when racial inequality in one domain bleeds into and is reinforced in another. Whereas structural racism refers to the deeply embedded inequalities within the structures of society, systemic racism emphasizes the interconnectedness and interdependence of various societal systems and institutions in perpetuating racial disparities.[32]

"What should we name our daughter?" I asked Luke in 2014. I was halfway through my pregnancy, and we had just learned we were having a girl. We knew from research that a person's name can affect how they're treated and the opportunities they encounter in life.

Within the employment sector, studies have consistently shown racial and gender disparities in hiring, promotion, and pay.[33] This unfair treatment begins before employers even meet the candidate. In 2004, two business professors published results of a field experiment in which they sent out 1,300 identical fake résumés to real job postings in Boston and Chicago. The résumés differed only in the names used, with researchers choosing the most common white and Black names given to children that year. Results showed that résumés with more common white-sounding names were more likely to get interview callbacks (10.6 percent) versus those with Black-sounding names (6.9 percent).[34] A more recent study by a team of economists sent out 83,000 fake résumés to 103 of the largest US employers in 2019. Findings showed not much had changed; on average, applications from candidates with a "Black name" got fewer callbacks than similar applications bearing a "white name."[35]

Within the education sector, disciplinary practices in schools disproportionately target students of color, resulting in higher suspension and expulsion rates among Black and Hispanic/Latino students compared to their white peers.[36] Standardized tests have been criticized for their cultural biases,[37] disadvantaging students from marginalized communities and perpetuating inequities in access to quality education and opportunities. Additionally, selection of which students are enrolled into advanced, honors, or Advanced Placement classes, or even go on to the next grade level, often favors students who are white.[38]

Within the criminal justice system, research consistently shows racial disparities in arrest rates, severity in sentencing outcomes, and incarceration rates,[39] highlighting the disproportionate impact of law enforcement policies and practices on people of color. Targeted marketing practices from businesses also perpetuate health inequities by promoting unhealthy products like tobacco,[40] alcohol, and unhealthy foods and beverages[41] in predominantly Black and Hispanic/Latino neighborhoods,[42] increasing risk for conditions such as obesity, heart disease, diabetes, and cancer. And, as covered in the previous chapter, racial disparities in health care treatment and access have been documented again and again. The disparate system of treatment that patients of color and other marginalized groups receive all predictably leads to poorer health outcomes. But because this is predictable, I also believe it is preventable.

The immensity of the task ahead, coupled with the weight of past research, can often feel overwhelming and demoralizing. Even while writing this chapter and the one before, I have had to step away multiple times to take a breath. As a public health expert who has seen the data and as a mom of multiracial children, I feel both a professional responsibility and a deeply personal commitment to do more than just discuss why racial disparities exist. I want to explore concrete solutions, leverage research, and collaborate with others on policies and programs that can create real change. My goal, shared by many in public health, medicine, social work, government, industry, and philanthropy, is to shift the status quo so that the inequalities we've seen for so long in the data are no longer the pattern for the future.

So what can we do about it?

We can target social determinants of health through evidence-backed policies and interventions, such as increased health care coverage, affordable housing initiatives, and reinvestment in marginalized communities. These show promise in reducing neighborhood, racial, and socioeconomic health disparities at their core by tackling the very roots of health and disease.

For instance, the Affordable Care Act's Medicaid expansion since 2014 has increased health insurance coverage for over 12 million people across 36 states; this added coverage reduced racial disparities in health care coverage, access, and health outcomes.[43] By providing affordable health care coverage to low-income individuals, these policies help remove barriers to accessing preventive care, screenings, and treatment for chronic conditions. This particularly helps people who are disproportionately uninsured or underinsured, including many people of color.

We can also promote initiatives for affordable housing. One study examined the impact of inclusionary zoning, a type of affordable housing policy, across hundreds of US jurisdictions. This policy promotes affordable housing and socioeconomic diversity by requiring developers to reserve a portion of new housing units for low- to moderate-income residents. Findings showed that in places with such policies, residents from all income levels had better heart health, including lower blood pressure, lower cholesterol, and lower rates of prescribed blood pressure medication, than those in places without such policies.[44] Such initiatives can also help address housing-related health disparities, such as overcrowding, substandard housing conditions, housing discrimination, and residential segregation. To minimize the impacts of gentrification, policies can prioritize affordable housing and anti-displacement measures. This includes protecting residents from eviction or displacement due to rising housing costs, supporting small businesses, preserving cultural heritage, and enhancing infrastructure, such as public transportation, schools, and health care, that benefits existing residents and strengthens community stability.

Additional policies that can reduce health disparities include fair access to vital resources like broadband internet and digital devices. Renewing federal programs like the Affordable Connectivity Program (ACP) can address the digital divide by providing a monthly broadband subsidy to eligible households and a onetime cash benefit to purchase a digital device.[45] Launched in December 2021 after the Bipartisan Infrastructure Law, the ACP provided support to over 23 million households until it ended on June 1, 2024.

Locally, cities like Fort Worth, Texas, partnered with Cisco to provide free Wi-Fi in areas with limited connectivity, benefiting tens of thousands of residents. Similarly, Charlotte, North Carolina, introduced Access Charlotte, a program providing free Spectrum Internet and Advanced Wi-Fi to over 5,000 households and 15 community spaces.[46] Other cities like Chattanooga in Tennessee and Loveland in Colorado are leading the way with community broadband networks.[47] These networks act as public internet service providers, offering affordable rates and competition with private companies to communities lacking internet access. And cities such as Sacramento; Seattle; Washington, DC; Harrisburg; and Boston rank among the top five in the nation by United Way for their efforts in digital equity.[48]

We can also make a stronger impact by investing in underresourced communities and promoting community-centered interventions that simultaneously tackle multiple social determinants of health. One example of an organization that has done this well on a local and national scale is the Green & Healthy Homes Initiative (GHHI).[49] Funded initially by the American Recovery and Reinvestment Act in 2009 under then vice president Biden, GHHI integrates public and private funds to create healthy, safe, and energy-efficient housing for low- and moderate-income communities across the US, including Tribal lands (territories held in trust by the federal government for the use and benefit of federally recognized American Indian/Native American Tribes). GHHI community sites are often in areas that experience high poverty rates and racial disparities, where families face housing-related health hazards like lead exposure, asthma triggers, and mold.

By improving the quality and energy efficiency of housing in underinvested neighborhoods, GHHI helps mitigate environmental health hazards and reduce the risk of respiratory illnesses, lead poisoning, and other health issues commonly linked with housing conditions, as well as reduce the cost of families' gas and electric bills. Their work has been shown to improve the health and well-being of residents in addition to reducing health care costs and absenteeism from school and work.[50] GHHI also focuses on skills training, job creation, and capacity building within the communities it invests in. By focusing on marginalized populations and addressing the root causes of health, like housing and employment, comprehensive initiatives like GHHI can play a crucial role in promoting health and economic opportunity.

Finally, it is critical to prioritize underserved communities when disasters are anticipated through coordinated national, state, and local level responses. Vulnerable populations, such as low-income families and communities of color, are disproportionately impacted by both natural disasters like hurricanes, floods, wildfires, and heat waves, as well as human-made disasters like chemical spills and water contamination. These communities suffer more due to preexisting socioeconomic disparities and limited access to resources. This was starkly evident in 2005, after Hurricane Katrina devastated New Orleans. Families in poorer, mostly Black neighborhoods bore the brunt of the damage and faced greater challenges in safely evacuating and rebuilding homes and communities.[51]

To enhance the ability of communities in historically marginalized areas to withstand and recover from disasters, we can implement and invest in proactive measures such as infrastructure strengthening, early warning systems, targeted evacuation and transportation plans, emergency supply distribution, neighborhood-based disaster response teams, and community-led efforts.[52] A review showed that targeted investments in flood-mitigation measures and infrastructure improvements in disadvantaged communities helped reduce the impact of flooding events and prevent long-term displacement.[53]

As I delved deeper into the research, I couldn't help but notice that most studies on neighborhood health disparities focused on cities or large counties. But in America and around the world, billions of people live, work, and play in vast rural areas, each with its own distinct characteristics, much like cities. I wondered: What stories do these communities hold? How do they weather the calm and the storm, and most importantly, what can we do better to support them?

CHAPTER 4

Living on the Margins

A good 1,311 miles away from Boston's cityscape and brick-lined streets, where Dunkin' coffee fuels the relentless traffic on I-93, is the quiet, sunbaked rural town of Panola, Alabama. Dorothy Oliver, a semi-retired sixty-eight-year-old Black woman, turned off her old, flickering TV with a heavy sigh. It was early March of 2020, and the world outside her tiny weathered general store was spiraling into chaos. The news had become a relentless whirlwind of warnings about a mysterious virus sweeping across the globe, each headline sounding more ominous. Dorothy gazed anxiously out at the streets of her town where the slow rhythmic pace had always been a comfort. Now, those same streets seemed to be on the brink of a gathering storm, one that she knew could be devastating.

The owner of the town's only general store, Dorothy felt a growing urgency to protect her community. She began ordering masks, hand sanitizer, and cleaning supplies, diligently stocking her store's shelves with essentials.[1] Her proactive measures contrasted with the general indifference of her neighbors. Just days earlier, a fellow church member had remarked to Dorothy, "I'm not sure what to make of it. . . . I'm not seeing anyone getting sick."

Their lack of concern troubled Dorothy even further. Nestled on the edge of Alabama and sharing a border with Mississippi, Panola epitomizes life on the margins. The town itself is a patchwork of modest, single-story homes, many of which have seen better days. The roads are mostly gravel and dirt, winding through the community like faded lines on a worn-out map. The conveniences of modern life are nowhere to be found—no grocery stores, pharmacies, shopping centers, schools, hospitals, or clinics. Dorothy's general store is one of the few hubs where locals gather to buy supplies, exchange news, share stories, and check on one another.

Despite its challenges, Panola radiates a comforting warmth. The town's sense of community is palpable and thick as the Alabama summer heat. With a tiny population of around four hundred, Panola is a predominantly Black community where residents have forged close-knit bonds that come from generations of living side by side. People know each other by name, and the church is a cornerstone, serving as a place of worship, social interaction, and mutual support. In a world that seems to grow more disconnected day by day, Panola's tight-knit friendships and mutual support are a rare and precious commodity.

Dorothy's deep-rooted love for her town propelled her into action, despite COVID-19 not yet having reached Panola's doorstep. Her concern was primarily driven by Panola's stark lack of infrastructure. As an unincorporated community, Panola does not have the local government that one might find in larger towns or cities. Instead of a mayor or city council, Panola's governance and public services are managed by officials in Sumter County, nearly thirty miles away. The lack of local administration means that residents routinely face challenges in getting essential services and advocating for vital resources. The closest health care facility is nearly forty miles away, a daunting distance for residents without reliable transportation. This extreme lack of infrastructure found in rural communities like Panola poses major challenges in normal times that become devastating during crises.

Years earlier, Panola's lack of health care access had taken a devastating toll on Dorothy. One evening, her husband was in a severe truck accident in Tuscaloosa, leaving him with critical injuries and severe damage to a major artery in his chest. The emergency medical responders, recognizing the gravity of his injuries, determined that he wouldn't survive the nearly two-hour ambulance ride to Birmingham, the closest city with the necessary tertiary care. So in Tuscaloosa he stayed, where he took his final breath.

"I truly believe that if we could have gotten my husband to Birmingham, he would have been okay," Dorothy said, her voice steady despite the deep grief shadowing her face.

In addition to being rural, Panola is low-income. Many families here do not own cars, relying instead on bicycles, shared rides, or even horses to get around. For these families, purchasing masks, hand sanitizer, or additional cleaning supplies to reduce the spread of COVID-19 were extravagances they could barely afford. Survival, day by day, remained the primary concern.

And, like hundreds of other rural communities across the US, Panola does not have broadband. Dorothy was one of the fortunate residents with Wi-Fi, and even she struggled with slow and spotty internet connections. This digital divide made it challenging to stay informed about the virus and secure basic necessities. The COVID-19 pandemic brought all these vulnerabilities into sharp focus, highlighting the gaps in health care access, transportation, economic stability, and digital connectivity that make life on the margins particularly precarious.

Frequently overlooked and underresourced, rural areas struggle with limited medical facilities and access to high-paying jobs, inadequate infrastructure, and higher poverty rates, making them especially vulnerable during public health disasters. According to the United States Department of Agriculture (USDA), over 46 million people (14 percent of the US population) lived in rural areas in 2022.[2] Data from the Federal Reserve's Survey of Consumer Finances indicate that the median net worth for rural households was $146,400 in 2022, while for urban households it was $199,200.[3] Rural communities are 76 percent non-Hispanic/Latino white and include significant, growing populations of Black, Hispanic/Latino, Native American, and other racial and ethnic groups.[4]

All rural areas experience significant economic challenges, with the US poverty rate in rural areas at 15.4 percent in 2019 compared to 11.9 percent in urban areas.[5] Geographically, rural communities span the entire country, from vast farmlands and small towns to remote regions. Many Tribal lands are located in rural areas, home to Indigenous populations who face unique challenges due to historical and systemic inequities, including forced displacement. These factors collectively exacerbate health crises within rural populations, underscoring the urgent need for targeted interventions and resource allocation.

Of the many challenges facing rural communities, among the most pressing is lack of adequate health care infrastructure and access. Research shows that rural areas have significantly fewer hospitals and health care facilities per capita compared to urban areas.[6] In fact, rural residents often travel more than twice as far as their urban counterparts to access care,[7] a distance that can mean the difference between life and death in emergencies, as Dorothy and her husband tragically experienced. The shortage of medical facilities also severely limits access to primary care and specialist services, contributing to higher rates of chronic diseases, disability, and preventable conditions like diabetes and heart disease in rural populations.[8]

Rural areas also struggle with shortages of health care professionals. The Health Resources and Services Administration designates many rural regions as Health Professional Shortage Areas (HPSAs). In 2020, rural regions had only 5.1 primary care physicians per 10,000 residents, compared to 8.0 in urban areas; 4.7 dentists per 10,000 in rural areas versus 7.6 in urban regions; and 11.1 nurse practitioners, physician assistants, and certified nurse midwives per 10,000 residents, while urban areas had 14.7.[9] This substantial shortage of health care professionals across a range of preventive, primary care, and specialty fields results in delayed diagnoses and treatments.

Recent trends are even more alarming. Since 2010, over 130 rural hospitals have closed,[10] with many more at risk of closure.[11] This trend exacerbates rural health disparities as medical services continue to disappear. In health emergencies, the lack of local hospitals means longer wait times for critical care, increasing mortality rates from conditions such as heart attacks, strokes, and traumatic injuries. A CDC report analyzing data from 2010 to 2022 found that rural Americans were more likely to die from heart disease, cancer, unintentional injuries, stroke, and chronic respiratory diseases before age 80 than their urban counterparts.[12] The report also revealed that preventable deaths were notably higher in rural areas, with nearly half (44 percent) of heart disease deaths among those under 80 deemed preventable, compared to 27 percent in urban areas. Additionally, over half of early deaths from unintentional injuries and chronic respiratory diseases in rural regions were preventable.

The inadequate health care infrastructure is further compounded by socioeconomic and transportation challenges. Research by the National

Rural Health Association highlights that more than one-third of rural adults report not getting needed medical care due to cost, compared to 18 percent of urban adults.[13] In addition, many rural residents lack access to or cannot afford private transportation and have scarce public transit options. This lack of reliable transportation can delay urgent and preventive medical care, resulting in greater reliance on emergency medical services, poorer health outcomes, and higher mortality rates compared to their urban counterparts.[14]

Though rural-urban health divides are seen across the globe, the US has greater geographical health disparities than several other high-income countries, including Canada, the United Kingdom, Australia, France, Germany, the Netherlands, New Zealand, Norway, Sweden, and Switzerland. As estimated by the 2020 Commonwealth Fund International Health Policy Survey, rural Americans are most likely to skip getting needed medical care due to cost than peers in other countries (36 percent in the US versus 14.4 percent in Canada as one example) and more likely to struggle with medical bills than their global peers (22.8 percent in the US versus 6.5 percent in Canada).[15]

Beyond health care, many rural residents live in food or pharmacy deserts that require them to travel long distances for fresh and nutritious food, prescription medications, over-the-counter drugs, and other essential health goods and services. The scarcity of healthy food options contributes to higher rates of obesity, diabetes, heart disease, and other diet-related health conditions in rural populations, while limited access to pharmacies makes it difficult to fill prescriptions and take medication.[16] Pharmacies are also access points for other critical health services, including routine immunizations, contraception prescriptions, and HIV prevention. According to the National Institute for Health Care Management Foundation, up to 80 percent of rural counties are designated as medically underserved areas, with pharmacy deserts a significant component of this designation.[17]

Service deserts in rural areas are the result of low population density and the financial challenges of sustaining grocery stores and pharmacies in low-demand locations. The unique geographical features of rural areas, such as mountains or large open spaces, also complicate the installation and maintenance of broadband infrastructure. Extending broadband infrastructure to these sparsely populated areas is expensive and often seen as unprofitable by private internet service providers.[18] Insufficient funding and policy support have also historically hindered efforts to close the broadband gap. About 22.3 percent of Americans in rural areas and 27.7 percent of those on Tribal lands lack broadband coverage, compared to only 1.5 percent of urban residents, as shown by data from the Federal Communications Commission (FCC).[19] The Pew Research Center reports that rural Americans also lag behind their urban counterparts in ownership of tablets, smartphones, and computer devices.[20]

The lack of broadband in rural areas obstructs access to up-to-date information, telemedicine, education, and economic opportunities, an experience Dorothy knew all too well. While she had sluggish and unreliable Wi-Fi, many of her neighbors had no internet access at all. This digital gap further isolated Panola during the pandemic, limiting the community's ability to protect itself, even when the long-awaited vaccine became publicly available.

The rollout of the COVID-19 vaccine occurred in late 2020 and early 2021. In larger cities, this was met with extensive media coverage, online registration systems, and vaccination sites. But in Panola, the story was starkly different. The town didn't even make it onto the initial list for vaccine disbursement—not a single mobile vaccine clinic was scheduled to visit. Dorothy knew this wasn't a mere logistic oversight; it was a dangerous, predictable gap that needed to be urgently addressed. Websites and registration portals provided information about where, why, or how to get vaccinated, but these were virtually useless in a community where Wi-Fi was a luxury, not a given.

Urban areas benefit from stronger infrastructure and greater access to information and resources because these advantages are driven and reinforced by an urban bias in health policies and funding mechanisms. Research shows that federal and state health care policies tend to prioritize urban populations, resulting in inequitable distribution of resources and services. For instance, a Kaiser Family Foundation report revealed that rural hospitals are more likely to face financial challenges and closures compared to urban hospitals, partly due to reimbursement policies that disadvantage rural providers.[21] During COVID, while urban hospitals were bolstered with national and state emergency funds and media coverage, rural hospitals were quietly shutting down, unable to keep up with the financial strain. As the pandemic unfolded, it became painfully clear that this urban bias skewed not just funding but media attention.

In the early months of the pandemic, Dorothy noticed how the media spotlight stayed on overwhelmed urban hospitals and cities devoid of life, while struggles in communities like hers went unnoticed. The narrative was clear: urban areas were the epicenters of the crisis, while rural areas were relegated to the background, barely a footnote in the national conversation. Studies show that rural regions receive less media coverage in general and especially during public health emergencies compared to suburban and urban areas, leading to a lack of awareness and resources to address their specific needs.[22] This lack of media visibility meant that critical response efforts were slow to reach places like Panola, and few seemed to care.

But Dorothy did, and she knew she couldn't afford to wait for distant help that might never come or might arrive too late. With policymakers and media outlets focusing their efforts elsewhere, Dorothy zeroed in on Panola. She tirelessly sourced essential protective and cleaning supplies for her community. As soon as the supplies arrived, she placed them front and center in her store and at checkout, making sure they were the first things her customers saw.

"Got your mask? Need some hand sanitizer? I got some more earlier this week," she would call out, her voice firm yet reassuring.

Each person who entered her store received a friendly reminder on the importance of protection and prevention, along with a personal conversation about how they were doing. Even behind her mask, her genuine concern and smile were evident through the crinkles around her eyes. With no vaccine or treatment in immediate sight, she was determined to prepare Panola for the impending storm, even if it felt like she was the only one standing guard.

"This area is majority Black. Kind of puts you on the back burner," Dorothy said matter-of-factly. "That's just it. I don't have to elaborate on that one."

Dorothy recognized the precarious situation facing her community, particularly with its predominantly Black population that endured historical and systemic economic, social, and political neglect. Her story illustrates how the combined effects of race, poverty, and living in a rural area intensify the difficulties faced by low-income, rural communities during disasters. Discriminatory policies like redlining and Jim Crow laws restricted Black communities' access to quality housing, education, employment opportunities, and health care. Similarly, Indigenous communities were often forcibly displaced to remote, rural areas with limited resources, creating long-standing economic disadvantages.[23] The geographic, economic, and social disparities are further compounded by political marginalization, leading to lower prioritization of rural communities for federal and state funding,[24] all of which lead to continued inadequate health care access, higher chronic disease rates, and shorter lifespans.[25]

COVID unleashed a storm that flooded the already fragile dam of rural health disparities. Studies revealed that rural communities across America bore a disproportionate burden of the virus, with higher rates of infection, hospitalization, and mortality compared to urban areas.[26] While rural areas are less densely populated, they have a higher proportion of residents aged 65 and older than urban areas[27] and are home to significant numbers of workers employed in industries such as agriculture, meatpacking, and manufacturing. These sectors often require close physical contact or frequent travel, thereby increasing the risk of infection and virus transmission.[28] The older population and higher rates of underlying health conditions in rural areas, combined with limited health care facilities, scarce resources, and inadequate testing infrastructure, further heightened rural America's susceptibility to the virus.[29] In March of 2020, Dorothy already sensed what lay ahead, long before the data confirmed it.

The moment she learned that a vaccine would be distributed, Dorothy dialed up her longtime friend and county commissioner, Drucilla Russ-Jackson. Together, they set on a mission to bring a mobile vaccine clinic to Panola. They hit the streets in Drucilla's trusty car, going door-to-door from the first light of the day until the fading glow of dusk, knocking on every household door. With each knock, Dorothy and Drucilla spoke personably and passionately about the vaccine, urging their neighbors to sign a petition. Their efforts didn't stop at doorsteps. At community meetings, Dorothy's voice rang with conviction as she stressed the importance of their collective action. She reached out to local officials, her determination visible in every conversation. Even her unreliable internet connection became an ally in her advocacy; she sent emails and made calls to state and city health departments to make sure Panola would not be forgotten.

———

But Dorothy needn't have been alone in championing for her community. Tackling rural health disparities demands a multifaceted approach that recognizes and prioritizes the distinct needs of these communities. Reliable broadband; well-staffed, equipped, and accessible health care facilities; dependable transportation; policies and media coverage that amplify rural voices; and emergency preparedness plans specifically tailored to the unique needs of rural communities. These elements are essential to close the gap and build healthy living conditions across every part of the country.

It's a priority to allocate funding for broadband access and improve digital infrastructure in rural areas. High-speed internet is essential for modern day-to-day living, facilitating remote work and schooling and access to banking and government resources. It allows us to connect with loved ones across vast distances and time zones, enables participation in social and community activities, offers a wealth of information and opportunities for personal and professional growth, and improves access to essential health resources and information, telemedicine and appointment scheduling, and remote consultations and follow-up care. High-speed internet isn't just a luxury—it's a lifeline. By prioritizing policies that invest in broadband in rural areas, we can help make sure that no community is left behind in the digital age.

Bridging the digital divide requires cooperation from all levels of government, alongside active partnership with industry, nonprofit organizations, and communities. At the national level, it's critical to revitalize the Affordable Connectivity Program, as discussed in chapter 3. Other bipartisan initiatives like the Digital Equity Act strive to ensure all communities have equal opportunities to participate digitally,[30] while the Accurate Map for Broadband Investment Act of 2023 aims to enhance broadband access by reallocating funds, using the latest National Broadband Map data that highlight areas in most need.[31]

State-level efforts also play an important role, with several states implementing initiatives to expand broadband access. In 2010, California established the Broadband Council, providing a platform for state agencies to collaborate, exchange information and insights, and propose policy measures to improve broadband accessibility in underserved areas.[32] Meanwhile, Minnesota set the pace with legislatively mandated broadband speed goals overseen by the Office of Broadband Development, complemented with a robust grant-matching program.[33] Maine became the first state to have its digital equity plan accepted by the Department of Commerce's National Telecommunications and Information Administration, with a strategy designed to tackle disparities in digital access, skills, and affordability statewide.[34]

Other policy initiatives include expanding health care services, particularly leveraging telemedicine and mobile clinics, alongside increased funding for essential supplies, staffing, and testing sites for rural areas. Telemedicine can be a transformative solution, reducing barriers of distance, transportation, and scheduling that often prevent rural patients from accessing distant health care facilities. Its versatility spans routine primary care, mental health counseling, chronic condition follow-ups, and more.[35] Additionally, mobile clinics serve as vital lifelines, delivering preventive care, screenings, and vaccinations directly to underserved rural communities. By expanding telemedicine and mobile clinic services, policymakers can better equip rural, low-income communities to navigate disease outbreaks while also improving their health, here and now.

To address the dire shortage of emergency and tertiary care for more severe injuries and conditions in rural areas, policymakers can offer robust financial incentives and support programs to help rural hospitals maintain essential emergency care services and to increase the number of rural emergency hospitals.[36] This includes supplying these facilities with adequate resources and staffing to proficiently handle critical cases. Furthermore, policymakers can establish coordinated regional emergency response networks, which empower rural hospitals to collaborate with larger medical centers for critical consultation, more seamless patient transfer, and effective resource coordination during crises. Directing resources to transportation infrastructure, including roads and air ambulance services, can also expedite and safeguard patient transfers from remote areas to hospitals equipped with higher levels of care.

Another important strategy to promote rural health is to invest in public health preparedness and emergency response.[37] Unfortunately, many rural areas are unequipped to handle emergencies like pandemics or natural disasters. By providing funding for emergency preparedness training, equipment, and resources, policymakers can enhance the capacity of rural communities to respond to and recover from health emergencies. This proactive approach can simultaneously reduce rural communities' vulnerability while improving resilience to future crises.

Ultimately, we must prioritize the social and structural determinants of health as a cornerstone to promote overall well-being in communities no matter their size or location.[38] Policies and programs that reduce poverty, enhance economic stability, and expand access to affordable housing and quality education can directly address the root causes of poor health. So can efforts to improve the physical, service, and social environments through creating safer, more accessible public spaces and infrastructure, investing in additional grocery stores, and developing green spaces. Addressing these root issues improves the health and longevity of rural residents, as well as sets the stage for a better future for communities everywhere.

In the downstream approach, we celebrate trailblazers like Dorothy who swim against the currents of structural inequities to effect change. The upstream approach, however, challenges us to reshape communities like Panola from their very foundations, tackling the root causes of poor health head-on. This approach urges us to shift from solely relying on individual endeavors toward the transformative task of building robust, fair systems. By strategically investing in policies and initiatives that acknowledge and elevate the distinct needs of rural regions, we can build and rebuild communities that can survive a storm and thrive in its wake.

CHAPTER 5

The Strength of Weak Ties

Nestled between Park Slope and Bay Ridge, two of New York City's wealthiest neighborhoods, lies Sunset Park, a vibrant middle-class enclave known for its breathtaking sunsets over the Manhattan skyline. Once an agricultural hub in the 1830s, Sunset Park evolved into an urban haven for immigrants throughout the twentieth and twenty-first centuries, becoming home to an ethnically diverse and lively community. Marielis's family, like many others, had immigrated from the Dominican Republic in the 1980s. The neighborhood thrived with people from Puerto Rico, Ecuador, Mexico, Colombia, and El Salvador, creating a rich tapestry of cultures.

Marielis's uncle was a familiar figure in Sunset Park. He took daily strolls from Fifty-Second Street to Fifty-Seventh, where Marielis's mom (his sister) lived on the first floor of a four-story Section 8 apartment building. They would exchange lighthearted jokes and neighborhood gossip through her kitchen window, his laughter echoing down the street. On his way back home, he often picked up a sandwich from the Dominican corner store.

"Lili, como tú ta?" he would call out every time Marielis was sitting by the kitchen window.

Standing at six foot one and around 250 pounds, Marielis's uncle had a larger-than-life presence. His full-body laughs were contagious, and he gave bear hugs powerful enough to knock the wind out of her. He taught Marielis to dance bachata and merengue as a child, infusing their family gatherings with joy and rhythm. Everyone in the neighborhood knew his name, not just for his size but for the open, community spirit he embodied.

At the peak of New York City's COVID surge in the spring of 2020, Marielis stayed connected with her mother, uncle, and grandmother (her mother and uncle's mom) through phone calls and texts. Her uncle's fiftieth birthday was approaching. He was the type who didn't want a fuss made over his own birthday but delighted in celebrating others'. The day came and went quietly, which was just as well—he'd been feeling off, with a sore throat, chest discomfort, and intermittent fevers. Marielis's grandmother made him a concoction of her ginger, onion, and cough medicine to take home.

On Friday, April 17, he felt well enough to pick up some cold and flu medicine from the local pharmacy. As usual, he stopped by Marielis's mother's kitchen window on his way home.

"Text me if you want to do something later," she called out.

"Another time," he replied, waving her off.

On the morning of Monday, April 20, Marielis was preparing breakfast for her niece and nephew when she received a frantic call from her sister. No one had seen their uncle since Friday. He wasn't responding to calls, texts, or knocks on his door either. Neighbors were complaining about the incessant noise from his TV, and the building superintendent called the police to assist with entering the studio apartment.

When Marielis, her sister, and their mother arrived, a sense of dread hung thick in the air. They pounded on his door, calling his name and desperately hoping for some kind of answer. When the superintendent finally unlocked the door, the apartment greeted them with an eerie quiet, save for the droning murmur of the television. As they stepped in, what met their eyes was a sight Marielis would never forget. Her uncle was lying on his stomach on his bed, dressed in his usual white, sleeveless undershirt, now stained and rumpled, with a flannel shirt thrown casually at the edge of the bed.

At the foot of the bed, his pristine white Nike Air Force 1s lay neatly side by side, as if he had carefully placed them there before collapsing. The remote control was wedged between his arm and his leg, and his phone lay right next to it, as if he had been in the middle of something before everything went wrong. Blood had crusted around his mouth and trailed down his swollen face, a painful testament to the lonely struggle he had endured in his final moments. Marielis stood frozen, the reality of the scene sinking in. Her uncle, who had always been the life of family gatherings, was now so still in this small, suffocating apartment.

As Marielis, her sister, and their mother stood in shock, the door creaked open further and the two policemen peered in, taking in the tragic scene before stepping back out into the hallway.

"Please state your name and relationship to the deceased," one requested, his voice firm but not unkind. Marielis's mother stood silent, her eyes glazed and her face blank. She did not utter a word and would not for days after.

"How many days has it been since you last heard from him?" the other policeman asked.

Marielis's mother remained silent. The questions kept coming.

"What's his race and ethnicity? His age? What did he do for a living? Was he sick? Did he have COVID? Had he recently picked up medicine from the pharmacy?"

With each question, the weight of the situation pressed down heavier on Marielis and her family. Finally, the dam broke. Her mother, who had held it together through the initial shock, started to bawl, her cries echoing through the small apartment and the hallway. It was the first time Marielis had ever seen her mother cry. The sight alone was heart wrenching, but the blue surgical mask covering her mother's face made it even more unbearable. Their grief crashed into them like a tidal wave, compounded by the immediate and brutal reality they now faced at the height of the pandemic.

It was now 1 p.m., and the police informed Marielis that if they didn't have burial plans for her uncle, he would be buried as a John Doe. Across the five boroughs of New York City that spring of 2020, funeral homes and morgues were over capacity. Each week's death toll seemed to shatter the previous week's. Bodies without designated arrangements were placed in wooden crates and buried in mass graves. Marielis and her family had until 5 p.m.

Panic set in, momentarily displacing grief. "What are we going to do?" Marielis thought. One of her aunts had a plot available, intended to be reserved for their still-living grandmother. But the plot was not fully paid off. To secure it for her uncle, they needed to come up with $1,100. And they still needed to find a funeral home to pick up her uncle's body and store it until they could bury him.

Marielis sprang into action, calling about thirty funeral homes across Brooklyn, Manhattan, Queens, and the Bronx. She called homes in every borough except Staten Island, where the convoluted bus system made it hard to reach without a car, unlike the reliable MTA trains in other boroughs. The conversations were the same: "Hello, are you picking up any bodies? Do you have space in your fridge? Are you doing cremations?"

Many funeral homes didn't answer. Others said no outright. Some questioned why she needed fridge space. Marielis didn't have the strength to explain after the fifth call. Finally, after what felt like an eternity, she found a funeral home on the opposite side of Brooklyn with available space. They agreed to pick up her uncle's body and hold it until arrangements could be finalized. Marielis promised to call them back, asking if they could save the space until she had secured the plot funds. The funeral home agreed, providing a glimmer of hope amid the chaos.

The next task loomed. With little in her family's bank accounts, Marielis knew she had just a few hours to raise $1,100 to ensure her uncle had a dignified burial—a place where they could visit, mourn, and honor his memory. On top of that, they needed an additional $500 in cash for the funeral home to come and pick up his body. If they failed, they would face the grim reality of city officials taking his body away in an unmarked pine box, alongside the hundreds of others piling up in New York City each day.

An aunt that was particularly close to Marielis's uncle emptied her savings account. Marielis herself contributed $200. It was a significant amount for her, as she had been saving every penny earned from her work-study job for her next semester's expenses at Boston University. But there was no question in her mind about the right choice. Despite contributions from close family members, they were hundreds of dollars short of their goal.

As Marielis stepped out of the building to speak with her sister, she was confronted by a scene that felt surreal. A crowd of mostly unfamiliar faces had gathered and formed a line, and the sheer number of people made her head spin. "Who are these people? Why are they here?" she wondered, feeling a mix of confusion and overwhelm.

Word had spread swiftly through their community about her uncle's sudden passing, and his network of friends, neighbors, and acquaintances had come to pay their respects. Marielis, who had known her uncle only in the context of family gatherings, was stunned by the outpouring of grief from so many. Though strangers to her, they were not strangers to him.

Timidly, she introduced herself and explained their financial predicament. She felt immense guilt, as everyone she knew in her neighborhood was struggling financially. Many were blue collar, shift, or contract workers who had been recently laid off, living off dwindling savings with no clear idea of when they might return to work. Yet, despite their own hardships, the people outside her uncle's apartment didn't hesitate to help. They reached into their pockets, contributing whatever they could spare. Marielis felt a lump rise in her throat as the envelope filled with cash. Through their combined efforts, they managed to gather the money needed.

The final task remained. The funeral home had made it clear they would provide only storage service and would not clean or prepare the body due to COVID concerns, so Marielis and her sister did the best they could, using baby wipes and paper towels to gently clean him themselves. Carefully, they dressed him in a collared shirt and khaki pants, washed his face, brushed his hair, and said a prayer.

Despite the overwhelming grief and turmoil of the day, Marielis felt a flicker of hope and gratitude. Their collective effort, aided by her uncle's humble yet strong network of community connections, had made it possible to honor his memory with a dignified farewell amid the chaos of the pandemic. She watched as the funeral home staff carried her uncle's body, wrapped in a black plastic bag, down the steps on a stretcher. Only then did she realize she had been holding her breath and finally exhaled.

The experience left an indelible mark on Marielis. It was a stark reminder of the fragility of life and the power of community bonds in times of crisis. Every day in 2020, Hispanic/Latino adults were twice as likely to die from COVID compared to whites, even after adjusting for age.[1] Tragically, Marielis's uncle belonged to the 45-to-54-year-old age bracket, where the Hispanic/Latino community faced a staggering sixfold increase in death rates than their white peers.

This harrowing chapter in Marielis's life underscores the critical importance of social connections and networks in shaping health, especially in times of challenges. It highlights the power of strong and weak ties, the role and function of social networks, and how the connections we cultivate with others can help us in life and after death.

———

Social networks are the web of connections we build with people throughout our lives. At the center of this web, individuals like Marielis's uncle have threads extending to family, friends, neighbors, classmates, colleagues, and acquaintances. Each thread in this web represents a distinct relationship, characterized by factors such as trust, intimacy, frequency of interaction, strength, reciprocity, and duration.[2] Structurally, a social network can be described by its size (the number of people a member is connected to), density (the degree of interconnectedness between members), and homogeneity (similarity among members in demographics, values, interests, and other shared characteristics). All these factors contribute to the web's overall strength and resilience, and the social networks we form significantly influence many aspects of our lives, including our well-being.

Decades of scientific study link social networks to health. In a landmark study, social epidemiologists found that people with more social connections had significantly lower mortality rates over a nine-year period compared to those with fewer.[3] Another large cohort study tracked over 32,000 male health professionals for four years.[4] At the beginning, none of the participants had heart disease. Over the course of the study, 511 participants died from heart-related conditions. The results showed that socially isolated men (those who were unmarried, had fewer than six friends or relatives, and weren't part of any community or church groups) had higher risk of developing heart disease and stroke and dying from these conditions. This risk persisted even after accounting for factors such as age, smoking, hypertension, alcohol intake, body mass index, parental history of heart attack, and physical activity. In contrast, men with robust social networks experienced lower mortality rates, not only from cardiovascular disease but also from accidents and suicides.

Other studies show that having strong social connections is associated with lower rates of depression and anxiety,[5] reduced inflammation,[6] improved health behaviors,[7] and better overall physical health and longevity.[8]

These findings underscore the critical role that social relationships and networks play in shaping how well and long we live.

But *how* exactly do social networks influence health? To answer this, we need to look beyond social networks' size and structure and understand their functions—the dynamic interactions and exchanges that occur between network members. Social networks fulfill several critical roles that directly impact our well-being: they provide social support, facilitate social influence and regulation, enable social engagement and participation, and serve as conduits to other people, services, and opportunities.

SOCIAL SUPPORT

Let's first delve into *social support*, which can take the form of emotional, informational, or instrumental support.[9] Emotional support, such as expressing empathy, love, trust, and care, provides reassurance, acceptance, and encouragement. This type of support strengthens our sense of security and belonging, helping us navigate life's challenges and transitions with greater resilience. Whether coping with job loss, illness, grief, divorce, or embracing life changes like moving, starting a new job, welcoming a family member, or celebrating milestones, emotional support fosters stability and connection. Research confirms that receiving emotional support can reduce psychological stress and anxiety, lower the risk of depression, and even benefit physical health by reducing blood pressure and heart rate.[10]

Imagine surviving a major health crisis. Now consider how a supportive network of friends and family might affect your recovery. Researchers investigated this scenario by studying nearly 200 men and women who were hospitalized after a heart attack.[11] Their findings were revealing: patients who had more sources of emotional support were significantly less likely to die in the six months after their heart attack, regardless of the attack's severity, other health conditions, or factors like smoking and blood pressure. Lack of emotional support, conversely, was linked to an increased risk of dying within six months.

Individuals within a network can also provide informational support— the sharing of advice, information, guidance, or feedback that helps individuals navigate life.[12] This form of support can be vital for managing health by helping individuals make informed decisions and increase their exposure to opportunities.[13] Access to accurate health information and specialist referrals through a supportive network can greatly improve treatment outcomes and well-being. Without adequate informational support, individuals may experience increased health risks due to lack of knowledge or misinformation.[14]

Informational support extends its benefits to other aspects of life like employment, education, and housing—key social determinants of health discussed in prior chapters. Timely insights into job openings and interview tips through one's network can substantially boost chances of landing a job.[15] This in turn can provide financial stability as well as access to health insurance, social status, and a sense of purpose and community. Lack of informational support can result in missed critical opportunities, highlighting how this seemingly indirect form of support can profoundly influence health.

Instrumental support, or practical support, consists of tangible help provided by others, including help with daily tasks, financial aid, and resource sharing. Examples include grocery shopping, meal preparation, provision of childcare, scheduling medical appointments, offering financial help during hardships, or giving a ride. Practical support eases stress by directly removing or lightening the load of tasks, especially during illness, recovery from events like surgery or childbirth, or when abilities decline in older adults. Research shows that receiving such support speeds up recovery times as well as lessens the overall impact of illness.[16]

Social support through our networks can profoundly influence health, but its impact depends on who provides support and how it's delivered. In one of my team's studies of over 600 adults, we examined both positive support for healthy eating and physical activity and "social undermining," such as ridicule, offering unhealthy foods, or other behaviors that derail progress toward health goals.[17] We found that verbal encouragement and shared activities, like exercising together, promoted healthy behaviors, while undermining actions, especially from family, hindered progress. Notably, support from friends and coworkers was linked to healthy weight maintenance over time, whereas family undermining, particularly around diet, contributed to weight gain.

There have also been consistent findings of gender differences in the type and level of support received from social networks and their impact on health.[18] For women with fewer resources, social networks can sometimes harm mental and physical health by adding stressful caregiving roles instead of reducing their burden. These studies show that social support is not inherently positive or negative but depends on dynamics and interactions within one's network. If one source of support, such as family, is not supportive of health goals or changes, one can find alternative sources of encouragement and accountability by turning to friends, coworkers, or a new social group.

I still think back to that day when Maria's mom comforted me and walked me home after I had been harassed. Her presence ensured I got home safely, and the kindness she offered has stayed with me ever since. This small gesture embodied both emotional and instrumental support, reminding me how even brief moments of care from those in our network can leave lasting imprints. Overall, emotional, informational, and instrumental support are all important for helping us manage stress, cope with life's challenges, and recover from illness.

SOCIAL INFLUENCE

Beyond providing support, social networks significantly influence health and health behaviors through *social influence and regulation*. Our network shapes our lifestyles profoundly through setting norms and expectations. For instance, if family members and friends prioritize fitness and healthy eating, individuals within these groups are more likely to adopt similar behaviors. Research shows that health behaviors like what we eat and drink, how much we move, and how much time we spend on social media and screens are often guided by the habits and norms of our social circle.[19] Conversely, when a network normalizes unhealthy behaviors such as smoking, substance use, excessive drinking, or unsafe sex practices, its members are more likely to adopt these detrimental practices.[20]

A compelling example of this dynamic emerged from a long-term health study that tracked over 12,000 US adults for more than three decades.[21] The research revealed a striking pattern: if one person became obese, their friends were 57 percent more likely to become obese too. This effect rippled outward, increasing the likelihood of obesity by 20 percent among friends of friends, and by 10 percent among friends of friends of friends, extending up to three degrees of separation within social networks. This phenomenon illustrates the powerful impact of social norms on our behaviors and health. If our close friends or family members gain weight, it can subtly recalibrate our sense of what is "normal," and we may unconsciously adapt our own eating, exercise, and sleep habits to align with changing norms.

Changes in health behaviors, both beneficial and harmful, can ripple through a social network, influencing others along the way. Using data from the same cohort of 12,000 US adults that demonstrated the social spread of obesity, researchers examined the behaviors of smokers when smokers in their network quit. They discovered that when a spouse quit smoking, their partner's likelihood of continuing to smoke dropped by 67 percent. If a sibling quit, it reduced their family members' chances of smoking by 25 percent. When a friend quit, it lowered the smoking rates in their social circle by 36 percent.[22]

Using fitness tracker data, MIT researchers examined the running and activity habits of 1.1 million people in a global social network, finding that exercise can also be contagious.[23] If a friend ran an extra kilometer, sped up their pace, or added time to their run, they inspire others to run further, faster, or longer as well. Similar patterns have been reported on the spread of drinking habits[24] and vaccine attitudes and uptake[25] within social networks. These studies demonstrate the dual role of peer pressure *and* peer possibility—the power of social networks to both reinforce conformity and inspire personal change based on the actions and feedback of others.

SOCIAL ENGAGEMENT

Social networks also play a pivotal role in promoting *social engagement and participation*. Participation in community groups such as local clubs, religious organizations, or hobby-based activities does more than fill our calendars—they meet a fundamental human need for connection and purpose. These interactions enhance cognitive function,[26] improve mental health, reduce stress, and are linked to increased longevity.[27] These benefits stem from the supportive community structures, regular social interactions, and sense of belonging and fulfillment that such groups provide.

The COVID-19 pandemic vividly demonstrated the critical importance of social engagement as lockdowns, closures, and social distancing measures disrupted daily interactions. Research during this period confirmed what was visibly unfolding: reduced social interaction led to increased loneliness and heightened stress, anxiety, and depressive symptoms.[28] These impacts were especially severe among children, adolescents, and young adults,[29] for whom social engagement is vital for developing social skills, self-esteem, and personal identity. The loss of routine face-to-face interactions and community activities—typically facilitated by schools and neighborhoods—severely disrupted these developmental processes.[30]

CONDUITS

Finally, social networks serve as *conduits*, spreading infectious diseases like the flu, sexually transmitted infections, and COVID-19 through person-to-person contact, as well as serving as channels for sharing valuable information and resources such as health care, housing, and job opportunities.

These conduits work through two types of connections, both of which are indispensable: strong ties and weak ties. Strong ties, exemplified by close relationships like that between Marielis and her uncle, provide readily available emotional and practical support. Weak ties—those connections with acquaintances, colleagues, and casual contacts—though less frequent and intimate, serve as bridges to different social circles,[31] enabling the flow of new information and opportunities not available within one's immediate network. This can lead to substantial health benefits, from accessing new health information to discovering job opportunities.

Marielis's uncle's weak ties played an unexpected but crucial role in securing the funds needed for his burial deposit. Despite the suddenness of the situation, his broader network quickly mobilized, demonstrating how weak ties can provide significant support during a crisis. Research shows that diverse networks of weak ties are linked to lower rates of depression and anxiety, greater success in job searches, and reduced mortality risk.[32] Both strong and weak ties serve as lifelines that provide the resources and support needed to navigate life.

Marielis's story of how weak ties can mobilize resources illustrates the broader concept of *social capital*—the collective strength and resilience of a social network and how well the web holds together when disaster strikes. It includes the level of interpersonal trust and norms of reciprocity and mutual aid between members, enabling access to support, information, resources, and opportunities.[33] When people within a community are more likely to trust each other and offer one another help, they strengthen the web, making it more reliable and supportive for everyone involved.

But not everyone has equal opportunity to build strong social capital. Structural factors such as income inequality can make it harder for communities to develop social trust, come together, and provide essential help during tough times.[34] Geography also plays a role. In remote areas like Dorothy's Panola, limited access to transportation, health care, and broadband can make it difficult to mobilize resources quickly in emergencies. Studies, however, demonstrate that rural communities may have more neighborhood social capital than urban counterparts,[35] possibly because rural residents may invest more time in cultivating strong relationships, given the fewer people and limited resources in less populated areas.

Historically, social capital was rooted in local communities in which trust and reciprocity thrived through close-knit networks like families, neighborhoods, and religious groups.[36] These bonds were foundational for mutual support, collective action, and cohesion. The rise of industrialization, urbanization, and globalization dramatically altered these dynamics, leading to a widespread decline in trust toward institutions and fellow citizens.[37] Social landscapes have further been fragmented because of widening economic inequality, political polarization, and rapid technological changes. While internet and social media provide tools to connect people across geographic borders and time zones, these modalities of communication and relationship-building fall short of the depth and authenticity provided through in-person interactions. But why is it important to revitalize trust in community and social networks, and how does this relate to health?

First, social capital fosters collective action and efficacy, empowering communities to tackle shared challenges, such as addressing rising rent prices, responding to new developments that impact their neighborhoods, or preparing for a winter storm. Second, social capital is pivotal in facilitating the diffusion of innovation—it helps spread new ideas, practices, and resources across networks, enhancing learning and adaptation within communities. Third, social capital bolsters informal social control, enabling community members to intervene when needed, such as addressing vandalism or collective adult supervision at playgrounds, pools, and parties. Last, the informal social interactions that form the bedrock of social capital, such as neighborly kindness and readiness to help strangers, cultivate a profound sense of solidarity and trust.

The power of social capital is especially evident during natural or human-made disasters, as demonstrated by the Chicago heat wave of July 1995. This devastating event claimed the lives of 739 individuals over a span of five scorching days, with heat indices soaring between 100 and 124 degrees Fahrenheit. Most victims were elderly residents of low-income neighborhoods who, lacking air conditioning, were reluctant to open windows or seek cooler environments outdoors due to neighborhood safety concerns. Analyses revealed a stark overlap between the geographic distribution of heat-related deaths and areas of concentrated poverty in the city.[38]

This tragic episode underscores the critical role of social support, social networks, and social capital in times of crisis. Neighborhoods in Chicago with stronger social ties and mutual aid networks were better equipped to check on vulnerable neighbors, share resources like cooling centers, and provide essential aid. In these communities, residents were more likely to trust one another, seek help, and accept support. In contrast, areas with weak social connections and poorer community cohesion struggled to cope with and recover from the heat wave's devastating impact. Given this, how can we build social capital in communities where it is lacking?

For communities with limited social capital and resources, building this vital asset involves establishing meaningful connections that enrich individual lives and strengthen communal bonds. Building social capital can take three forms: bonding, bridging, and linking.[39]

Bonding social capital involves deepening supportive relationships within groups that share similar backgrounds or interests. For instance, local community fairs, new parent groups, and annual block parties strengthen bonds among group members, creating a sense of security and support. *Bridging social capital* extends beyond immediate social circles to connect individuals across diverse social groups. One example would be a community center that hosts multicultural festivals, encouraging interactions and understanding between different cultural groups within the same town or city. *Linking social capital* connects individuals and communities with those in positions of power or who have access to significant resources. This can be seen in community advocacy groups that partner with local government officials to secure funding for community projects or to influence policy decisions that benefit their community.

Consider Hurricane Katrina, one of the deadliest natural disasters in US history. Striking the Gulf Coast in August 2005, the hurricane unleashed catastrophic flooding across New Orleans, Louisiana. The devastation resulted in extensive infrastructure damage, displaced thousands, and caused over 1,800 deaths. The impacts were most severe in Black, low-income, and historically redlined communities.[40] Due to structural racism and income inequality, social capital was unevenly distributed by race and class, leading to inequities in who could escape the storm.[41] For instance, many Black, low-income families in New Orleans lacked a car, making it near impossible to follow evacuation orders.

Researchers conducted an in-depth analysis of forty families during and after the hurricane, revealing that residents, particularly those with low incomes, depended on, built, and sometimes exhausted all forms of social capital for individual, family, and community survival.[42] *Bonding social capital* allowed families to coordinate with each other on emergency and evacuation plans, demonstrating the strength of tight-knit, familiar relationships in moments of urgent need. As the hurricane devastated communities across zip code, socioeconomic status, and race, *bridging social capital* became essential to facilitate the receipt and provision of aid across sociodemographic lines, highlighting the importance of inclusive networks that extend beyond one's immediate social circle during crises. *Linking social capital* connected families with policymakers, government entities, nonprofit organizations, and advocacy groups that helped victims access critical resources, illustrating how strategic relationships can mobilize support. These lessons from Hurricane Katrina illustrate how social connections—whether within close communities, across broader societal divisions, or through influential networks—play indispensable roles in navigating the immediate challenges of a disaster and rebuilding lives and communities in the long term.

Building robust social networks rich in social capital, particularly in underserved communities, requires thoughtful, targeted strategies. Research suggests several key approaches that foster social interaction, trust building, and community engagement.

One approach is to implement community-based planning and programming that encourages local participation and new interactions, which can significantly boost social cohesion.[43] To build a sense of shared purpose and mutual reliance, community activities can empower and engage community members in decision-making to shape their environments, whether through community gardens, local sports leagues, or celebrations that bring residents together.

Also critical is infrastructure development, as members of a community are more likely to connect with others when supported by their physical environment. This can take the form of enhancing public spaces such as parks, libraries, and community centers, which provide accessible, safe, and vibrant social hubs and promote gatherings that increase daily interactions and build trust.[44] Urban planning and architecture can enhance this dynamic[45] by increasing walkability and creating mixed-use developments that combine residential, commercial, and recreational spaces. These developments often facilitate spontaneous social encounters, enriching community ties.

Yet another approach is the expansion of programs that promote volunteering and civic participation, empowering residents to take active roles in their community's development. This in turn strengthens community ties and trust among members. Studies show that communities with active volunteer networks exhibit higher levels of trust and civic engagement, facilitating stronger social connections across diverse groups.[46]

At the policy level, governments and local authorities can enhance community cohesion through targeted policies, such as subsidies for community projects, grants for local nonprofits, and support for cooperative business ventures. These policies can significantly strengthen both the economic and social fabric of a community.[47] Additionally, policies can focus on promoting work-life balance, like enhancing job flexibility; this raises social capital by increasing members' capacity to engage in their community and invest in personal relationships.[48]

Communities can further strengthen social capital by strategically leveraging technology.[49] This can involve digital platforms that facilitate community discussions, service exchanges, or local event promotions, connecting members to a larger community. Neighborhood-based apps, for instance, help build local ties by allowing neighbors to share resources, exchange services, and stay informed about local events and issues.

Social media platforms, on a larger scale, can be powerful tools for mobilizing resources, raising awareness, and uniting communities around common causes. During the 2020 Australian wildfires, comedian Celeste Barber's Facebook campaign mobilized over a million people worldwide, raising $51 million for relief efforts.[50] Similarly, the Ice Bucket Challenge went viral, boosting global awareness and generating $115 million in funding for amyotrophic lateral sclerosis (ALS) research.[51] Participants filmed themselves pouring ice water over their heads and challenged others to do the same or donate to ALS research, showcasing the power of social media as a tool for fundraising and advocacy.

Our social connections are more than just a source of companionship—they are powerful drivers of our health and resilience, influencing our lives individually and collectively. The enduring impact of the social ties of Marielis's uncle, whose network provided crucial support in the days after his death, vividly demonstrates how the relationships we nurture can sustain and help us throughout life and beyond.

CHAPTER 6

What's in a Name?

Say the word "Wuhan," and what comes to mind? For many outside China, it might conjure images of an authoritarian government or the birthplace of COVID-19. But not for me. Born in Wuhan in the 1980s, I immigrated to the US with my mother when I was nearly four to join my father in Boston, where we later became naturalized US citizens. To me, Wuhan is a city of memories.

It's the sounds of crickets chirping on hot, sticky summer nights, when my mother and I would drag our mats to sleep outside, seeking relief under the stars from the suffocating heat inside our small apartment. It's the sight of my breath fogging up the winter air as I shuffled to the kitchen for breakfast, bundled in four layers, where my mother would hand me a steaming bun, and I'd try to guess if it was sweet or savory before I took the first bite. My toddler years were filled with cousins' laughter and neighbors' chatter echoing down narrow hallways and open streets, my aunts' teasing and chiding voices, and the tight, enveloping hugs of my Nai Nai (paternal grandmother), her floral-print blouses faintly scented with green tea and lotion.

These were fond memories I shared with others, moments that connected me to my past. But in 2020, for the first time in my life, I stopped sharing that part of myself.

December 31, 2019, was quieter than the previous fourteen New Year's Eves that Luke and I had shared. Normally, we'd pick a festive restaurant, toast with friends, and stay out late. But with much travel planned for

2020, we opted for a cozy night in with our daughters, then ages five and nearly three. After the girls drifted off to sleep, we popped open a bottle of prosecco and watched a movie. At midnight, we called and texted family and friends.

"Xin nian kuai le!" I messaged my parents and brother.

The next morning, I called my dad. "How is everyone back in Wuhan? How is Nai Nai?"

"They're doing fine," he replied, but his voice carried a trace of sadness. "Grandma's memory isn't what it used to be."

We made plans to have dinner at my parents' house for Chinese New Year later in January. Everything was as usual. As Luke and I curled up in bed, blissfully unaware, I couldn't have known that on the other side of the world, my birthplace was about to change forever.

That same day, Wuhan authorities confirmed to the media that they were investigating a mysterious illness.[1] By January 8, 2020, the *New York Times* reported that China had identified a new virus causing pneumonia-like symptoms.[2] On Chinese New Year, when we gathered at my parents' house to ring in the Year of the Rat, the virus crept into our conversation.

"They've canceled the festivities in Beijing," my dad said, his face clouded with unease.

Luke's eyebrows shot up. "Wow. That's a big deal."

It was. Chinese New Year is like Thanksgiving, Christmas, and New Year's rolled into one—a massive, weeks-long festival of reunions, red envelopes stuffed with crisp bills, endless dishes spread across tables, and the Spring Festival Gala, a variety show broadcast on the eve of the new year, lighting up every TV. This massive holiday is usually accompanied by an equally mammoth travel rush, typically from mid-January to late February, as students and workers in China travel back to their hometowns for family reunions or to go on vacation. The cancellation of festivities was a seismic shift.

"Most things are shut down in Wuhan," my mom said in a hushed voice. "They're in lockdown. You have to stay in your apartment. Prices for food and basics have doubled."

The lockdown in Wuhan had begun two days earlier, on January 23, 2020.[3] In the dead of night, at 2 a.m., notices pinged on smartphones, warning that by 10 a.m., public transit, airports, and highways would shut down. Wuhan, in central China, is a major national and international transportation hub. It was hard for me to imagine stillness and silence in a city that rivals the pace and noise of New York City. Travel restrictions were soon imposed on all the other fifteen cities in the Hubei province, home to fifty-seven million people.

I thought of the small apartments my aunts, uncles, and cousins live in. With eleven million residents (roughly the equivalent of New York City and Chicago combined), apartment buildings and complexes reign supreme in Wuhan—there are no single-family homes with basements, multiple floors, or backyards to escape to.

"How long will it last?" I asked, my stomach twisting.

His normally furrowed brow deepening with worry, my dad said, "No one knows."

A week later, on a cold, gray Friday in Boston, Wuhan surfaced in conversation at my department meeting. Usually, no one outside my family even recognized the city by name. But now, Wuhan was everywhere. I shared updates from my parents and described the stark reality of lockdown in a large city.

"Tell us how we can help," a well-meaning colleague offered. The unforgiving fluorescent light seemed to amplify the mixture of curiosity, concern, fear, and pity in the room. The conversation soon turned toward anti-Asian racism and reports of Asian people being harassed in public transit in Europe. Already in the first month of 2020, memes were circulating of people wearing hazmat suits standing over a bowl of noodles. How quickly it spreads.

For years, I'd introduced myself to students with a slide showing a map of China, a bright red circle over Wuhan. I shared with them my story about immigrating to Boston as a child and how my experiences as a busing student shaped my passion for public health. It was a piece of my identity I enjoyed sharing. But in the winter of 2020, as I prepared my lecture for a new cohort of students, I hesitated. My cursor hovered over the slide with the map of China. Then, I deleted it.

"It's not relevant," I told myself. "I'm not teaching a class on immigration or identity." I didn't speak of my immigrant story and birthplace to anyone for another two years.

The truth was, I hoped that omitting my birthplace from my story might shield me from the growing wave of anti-Asian sentiment. Maybe not telling people would make people not see. Except that everyone could see the espresso-black hair framing my face, the golden undertones of my light skin that deepens during the summer months, and the dark cocoa almond eyes shaped by my heritage. Features that loudly declared: ASIAN, NOT WHITE.

In the months that followed, I watched the word "Wuhan" flash across daily headlines, solidifying itself in the global imagination as the origin of COVID-19 and becoming a household word interchangeable with COVID. My birthplace became a red siren of danger, reduced to a caricature of fear, suspicion, and derision. To me, Wuhan was still home to my Nai Nai, uncles, aunts, and cousins. But to the world, it became something else entirely.

———

Disease has long been used as a tool to ascribe otherness and justify exclusion and maltreatment. During the early months of the COVID-19 pandemic, the Trump administration faced criticism for downplaying critical warning signs and focusing its messaging on the virus's geographic origins. Referring to COVID-19 as the "China virus," "Wuhan virus," or "kung-flu virus," the administration's language repeated a centuries-old pattern of scapegoating marginalized groups during outbreaks of contagion. This rhetoric directly contradicted the efforts of scientists, world leaders, and organizations like the World Health Organization, which sought to avoid stigmatizing language precisely to prevent the spread of fear, xenophobia, and discrimination.

Neither anti-Asian racism nor conflating specific racial or ethnic groups with a disease is new. As far back as the fourteenth century, records tell a recurring story: During infectious disease outbreaks, marginalized populations—already burdened by poor living conditions, limited access to medical care, and poorer health outcomes—became scapegoats. In the chaos of an outbreak, when death feels imminent and the mechanisms of disease and its remedies remain unknown, fear and misinformation often spread faster than the disease itself. This toxic combination of fear and misinformation fuels existing structural, social, and economic inequities, deepening the crisis and its impacts.

The Black Plague, or bubonic plague, remains the deadliest pandemic in recorded history, claiming an estimated 75–200 million lives globally and wiping out 30–60 percent of Europe's population between 1346 and 1352.[4] Today, we understand that the plague was caused by bacteria that likely spread from rodents to humans via infected flea bites. During the pandemic, however, Europeans across all socioeconomic classes scapegoated Jewish communities, falsely accusing them of spreading the disease by poisoning wells and food.[5] These accusations were rooted in long-standing antisemitic fears that Jewish presence threatened Christian rule in Europe. As the death toll rose, so did antisemitism, leading to widespread destruction of property and violent "retaliation" against Jewish residents. Massacres of Jewish communities began in Toulon, France, in 1348 and soon spread to Spain, Germany, and Switzerland.[6]

In January 1349, an enraged mob in Basel targeted the Jewish community, forcibly separating children from their parents. The children were baptized against their will, while the adults were taken to a wooden structure on an island in the Rhine and burned alive.[7] The violence escalated across Europe: in Strasbourg, where the Black Plague had not yet arrived, several hundred Jews were publicly burned alive on February 14, 1349, with the remaining Jewish community expelled from the city.[8] Elsewhere in Europe, Jews were persecuted through forced conversion to Christianity, expulsion from their hometowns, or murder. Authorities often stood by or actively participated in these attacks. By 1351, a wave of anti-Jewish pogroms (organized violent attack against a particular ethnic group, in particular Jews) had been documented, with the pogroms resulting in the destruction of hundreds of Jewish communities across Europe.

At the time of the Black Plague, germ theory, which proposes that certain diseases are caused by microorganisms too small for the eye to see,[9] had not yet been conceived. Over two hundred years later, aided with the invention of the microscope, Dutch scientist Antoni van Leeuwenhoek documented bacteria for the first time in 1676.[10] Another 216 years passed before Russian botanist Dmitri Ivanovsky discovered the tobacco mosaic virus in 1892, observing that infected plant extracts remained infectious even after passing through porcelain filters designed to trap bacteria.[11] Ivanovsky and Dutch microbiologist Martinus Beijerinck are credited with codiscovering this new category of infectious agents at the end of the nineteenth century,[12] which Beijerinck named *Contagium vivum fluidum* (Latin for "contagious living fluid").

These breakthroughs transformed our understanding of the nature of infectious diseases, how they were spread, and how they could be treated. The twentieth century brought the invention of antibiotics and vaccines, revolutionizing our ability to prevent and manage epidemics.[13] Despite these advances in science and medicine, the xenophobia that surfaces during public health crises has remained strikingly persistent. Derived from the Greek roots *xenos* (foreigner, outsider) and *phobos* (fear), xenophobia—fear of "the other"—continues to shape societal responses to crises.

The 1918–1920 influenza pandemic was the deadliest of the twentieth century, leading to at least fifty million deaths worldwide.[14] Like many of my peers, I first learned about this catastrophe in high school as the "Spanish flu." Yet the name is a misnomer, a by-product of how pandemics often amplify othering and blame. Scholars and historians agree that the virus most likely originated from avian flu in France, and at the time, Spanish newspapers referred to it as the "French Flu."[15] The term "Spanish flu" gained traction after Madrid's *ABC* newspaper published a headline on May 22, 1918, describing a mysterious illness spreading in Spain.[16] At the time, the world was reeling from World War I, and major nations, including the United States, imposed strict censorship to protect morale and prevent sensitive information from reaching enemy nations. Spain, a neutral country, became one of the few to openly report on the disease, unintentionally casting itself as the face of the pandemic. With little reporting elsewhere, the spotlight landed on Spain to take the blame.

But Spain wasn't the only target. In Senegal, it was called the "Brazilian flu." Brazilians blamed the Germans, Poles pointed fingers at the Bolsheviks, and Persians held responsible the British.[17] Across the globe, the pandemic's origin became a reflection of geopolitical tensions, with each nation casting suspicion on an outsider. Despite clear evidence that the virus neither originated nor spread from Spain, the pandemic is still widely remembered as the "Spanish flu," a lasting reminder of how misinformation and blame can shape collective memory.

This same pattern resurfaced in the early years of the COVID-19 pandemic. By doing so, it reignited anti-Asian sentiments that have long simmered in US history, fueling a surge in attacks, discrimination, and violence against Asian communities.[18] The roots of such xenophobia run deep in US history: the Chinese Exclusion Act of 1882 prohibited all Chinese immigration, legitimizing white violence against Chinese people and fostering racist media narratives about the so-called "yellow peril."[19] After a bubonic plague outbreak in San Francisco's Chinatown in the early twentieth century, authorities quarantined the entire neighborhood, blaming Chinese residents for the disease's arrival.[20]

Even after the repeal of the Chinese Exclusion Act in 1943, discrimination and violence persisted against Asians in the United States, from the US government's Japanese internment camps of WWII,[21] to anti-Vietnamese vigilantism by the Ku Klux Klan in Texas in 1979,[22] to the killing of Vincent Chin, a Chinese American, in Detroit in 1982 by two white men (a Chrysler auto-plant supervisor and his laid-off stepson) who blamed Chin for the success of Japanese auto imports and the subsequent loss of American manufacturing jobs.[23]

In more recent memory, public figures and media outlets continued to blame marginalized groups for major health crises: the HIV/AIDS epidemic of the 1980s was tied to Haitian Americans and gay men, the 2003 SARS epidemic to Asians, and the 2009 H1N1 epidemic to Mexicans. Both SARS and H1N1 fueled a surge of anti-immigrant sentiment. The first known case of SARS, an airborne respiratory illness caused by a coronavirus, was reported in Guangdong, China, in February 2003 and quickly spread to Hong Kong, Vietnam, Canada, and beyond.[24] While scientists raced to understand its cause and transmission, media coverage stoked fear, amplifying an us-versus-them narrative that associated Chinese people and culture with the disease.[25]

Public resentment and xenophobia surged. In the US, Chinatowns and Asian restaurants watched their revenues drop as fear and prejudice drove customers away.[26] The World Health Organization reported a total of 8,098 SARS cases globally during the outbreak, with 774 deaths.[27] Experts in retrospect weighed the stigmatization of the Asian community during SARS against the actual disease impact, and they deemed SARS an epidemic of fear rather than of disease.

The narrative surrounding the novel H1N1 virus, first detected in April 2009 near pig farms in Mexico, quickly became racialized.[28] Media outlets and commentators used harmful stereotypes to vilify Mexicans, with terms like "fajita flu"[29] and "the Mexican flu"[30] gaining traction. Mexican nationals and products from Mexico were widely shunned, reflecting how prejudice can ripple beyond individuals to entire economies. Stigma surrounding H1N1 also created barriers to care,[31] as Mexican Americans, fearing discrimination, were less likely to seek medical attention when ill,[32] further exacerbating the virus's spread. The rhetoric surrounding H1N1 and many other prior pandemics, like the "China virus" during COVID-19, highlights a painfully predictable pattern of using fears to scapegoat marginalized communities and amplify harm.

The first time I heard the terms "Wuhan virus" and "China virus" in a newsclip, I reflexively shut my laptop, as if I could shut out the visceral wave of emotion those words triggered. But I couldn't. They distorted everything Wuhan means to me—my memories, my heritage, and the humanity of the people who live there. I felt small, angry, fearful, and helpless. In the weeks and months that followed, at times I couldn't even bring myself to look in the mirror. The reflection staring back felt unfamiliar, burdened by a weight I didn't choose but couldn't escape. The weight of knowing that to some, my features are not a marker of heritage but a target. Each glance in the mirror felt like a confrontation: with the fear of being othered, the frustration at being misunderstood, and the guilt for feeling this way at all. How did I get to the point of wanting to hide what has always defined me?

The hatred and violence that followed were no surprise. I felt it brewing: the dual fear of rising anti-Asian sentiment and the growing threat of COVID-19 reflected in the eyes of familiar faces and strangers alike. Fear, history teaches us, is as contagious as any virus. Still, I clung to optimism. *Maybe it won't be that bad*, I told myself. I threw my energy into research and teaching and tried to drown out the headlines swirling across social media.

But as 2020 wore on, the reality became impossible to ignore. COVID-19 cases in the US continued to rise, testing remained woefully inadequate, and the pandemic narrative in the US and Europe persisted in scapegoating, shaming, and othering people from Wuhan and China—people like me. This rhetoric had devastating real-world consequences: by the end of 2020, anti-Asian hate crimes in the US had surged by 149 percent, according to the Center for the Study of Hate and Extremism.[33] Headlines were dominated by reports of verbal harassment, physical assaults, and violence targeting Asian Americans, painting a grim picture of escalating hate. One of the most tragic incidents was the deadly spa shootings in Atlanta in March 2021, where a gunman killed eight people, including six Asian women. Between March 2020 and March 2022, organizations like Stop AAPI Hate documented over 11,000 incidents of harassment, assault, and violence targeting Asian Americans.

While COVID-19 repeated historical patterns of scapegoating, it also exposed the contradictions of another harmful narrative: the model minority stereotype. This myth, which paints Asian Americans as universally successful and self-sufficient, masks the very real systemic and day-to-day economic, social, and health struggles faced by many in the community. It creates a paradox: we are cast as threats while simultaneously rendered invisible in conversations about opportunity, representation, and justice.

Within the broad Asian American category, the experiences of smaller subgroups bring to light significant disparities that debunk the model minority stereotype.[34] For example, only 23 percent of Hmong and Burmese adults in the US hold a bachelor's degree or higher, compared to 75 percent of Indian Americans, 54 percent of Asian Americans overall, and 36 percent of the general US population in 2019.[35] Income levels also vary widely, with the median annual household income for Burmese Americans at $44,400 in 2019, far below the $85,800 median for all Asian Americans.[36] And, as we've uncovered in prior chapters, educational and economic disparities translate into health divides, with Burmese Americans experiencing poorer health than East Asian groups that have also historically received more attention in health research.[37]

A closer look at the data also dispels the myth that Asian Americans do not experience health disparities. For instance, Asian Americans have the highest rates of undiagnosed diabetes among racial and ethnic groups, with studies estimating that over 50 percent of Asian Americans with diabetes remain unaware of their condition.[38] They are also the only racial or ethnic group in the US where cancer, not heart disease, is the leading cause of death among men and women.[39] Asian Americans have disproportionally high rates of cervical, liver, nasopharyngeal, and stomach cancers than other racial and ethnic groups.[40] Breaking down health data by specific subgroups reveals further disparities. Among women who have never smoked, 79 percent of lung cancer diagnoses occur among Chinese Americans, compared to 53 percent for Filipina Americans, 24 percent for Japanese Americans, 38 percent for Hispanic/Latinos, 21 percent for non-Hispanic/Latino whites, 15 percent for Native Hawaiians, and 14 percent for Black women.[41] These cancer patterns differ significantly from those seen in Asian countries, underscoring the unique health challenges Asian Americans face in the US.

Researchers also report that, alarmingly, anti-Asian discrimination can worsen cancer risks by driving tobacco use and weight gain while discouraging seeking cancer screenings or other essential health care services.[42] Asian Americans have also reported significantly higher levels of anxiety, depression, and post-traumatic stress as hate crimes and public stigmatization escalated post-COVID.[43] Yet, they remain among the least likely to access mental health services due to cultural stigma, language barriers, inadequate access, and lack of culturally competent care.[44] The model minority stereotype isn't a badge of honor; it's a major source of stress and a barrier to care.[45]

To tackle health disparities among Asian Americans, strategies must dismantle structural and cultural barriers. A first step is to collect more detailed racial and ethnic data. Asians in the US include over 21 distinct racial and ethnic groups who speak 23 languages that originate from Asia.[46] Yet they are often grouped into a single racial category and often combined with Native Hawaiian and Pacific Islander populations. Combining or averaging data in ways that obscure important information is a form of *aggregation or ecological bias*.[47] This practice hinders efforts in identifying, understanding, and addressing health disparities for groups with unique ancestral origins, histories, cultures, experiences, and needs.

Health programs and initiatives can be more effective by breaking down these categories, increasing Asian American representation and funding in health research, and improving access to screenings for health concerns like diabetes, cancer, and mental health.[48] Equally critical is expanding and training multilingual providers and culturally adapted therapies to address the challenges faced by this population. Public health campaigns can further normalize help-seeking behaviors by crafting targeted messages that respect cultural values and reflect the specific needs of individual subgroups.

Improving the health of Asian Americans—as with any community that faces stigma—begins with the words we choose. A simple yet powerful step anyone can take is to use neutral terms when describing health and disease, avoiding language that fuels stigma and discrimination. Patterns may be built by many and repeated over time, but it takes only one person to start a change.

As a public health expert who studies health and human behavior, I understand that people often resort to xenophobic language, imagery, and actions during crises as a way of managing fear and asserting power. Blaming others provides a temporary release from discomfort, a fleeting illusion of control in the face of chaos. But as someone in the stigmatized group, I found that my coping mechanisms (hiding and denial) were tenuous at best. I buried my birthplace and avoided drawing attention to myself, hoping to shield my family and myself from harm. But the more I tried to distance myself from my identity, the more I felt the weight of erasure. How long could I keep this up?

It wasn't until years later, at an Indigenous Moondance ceremony I attended in 2024, that I discovered that embracing heritage and confronting the trauma of erasure could lead to healing, not only for myself but for many communities that have endured such loss.

CHAPTER 7

The Other Side

In the town of Manchaca, Texas, where expansive fields meet endless skies, Abuela Rosa Tupina Yaotonalcuauhtli stands as a living bridge between past and present. As a licensed clinical social worker and healer, Abuela Tupina is deeply rooted in the Mexica traditions of her ancestors. Originating from the Valley of Mexico, the Mexica were Nahuatl-speaking people who once ruled the formidable Triple Alliance, better known today as the Aztec Empire.[1] Abuela Tupina's work takes rich threads of ancient healing practices, handed down through generations, and intricately weaves them together with modern techniques like cognitive behavioral therapy. This blend creates a vibrant, living tapestry that intertwines history, culture, spirituality, community, nature, and science.

The year 2020 unraveled many of these threads. In the span of two months, loss after loss frayed Abuela Tupina's life.[2] The tear began with the death of her sister from COVID-19, followed in quick succession by the deaths of her aunt, cousin, and sister-in-law. Each premature death was a stitch undone, ripping holes in the world Abuela Tupina knew and had helped craft.

These were personal family losses as well as communal catastrophes. The individuals she mourned were custodians of Indigenous oral history, culture, and language, each holding stories and traditions passed through generations. Their ancestors had lived for centuries on what is now known as the US–Mexico border, long before Spanish conquistadors invaded and colonized the Aztec Empire and before modern governments etched borders into the land. Her family members' passings, along with countless

Indigenous lives lost in the US, Canada, Mexico, Brazil, New Zealand, and Australia during the initial years of the pandemic, severed cultural lifelines that had connected and sustained their identities and communities across millennia.[3]

Abuela Tupina's childhood unfolded in the 1960s in a mining village in Ávalos, a small village in the northern state of Chihuahua, Mexico. Her village was also the site of a US smelting company, where workers endured long hours, low wages, and unsafe conditions, and toxic by-products contaminated the soil and water. Miners and farmworkers, cloaked in dust, trudged through the streets as they went about their daily grind. The village had no running water, depending on communal wells that seldom met its residents' needs. She wandered barefoot through the dusty paths and humble cement-block houses, her young mind often lost in thought as she navigated the rough terrain. Her village was a mosaic of hardworking families, all striving to carve out a better future from the harsh brown landscape.

Despite the pervasive poverty, the village thrummed with a strong sense of community and culture. Here, every face was familiar, and each person a vital thread woven into the fabric of daily life, tightly interlaced by shared history, present struggles, and dreams of a better future.

Each year, a group of unfamiliar white women visited around December 25, which always puzzled young Tupina. While she welcomed the novelty of seeing new faces in her village, she found their presence curious and out of sync with her community's traditions. Her village celebrated on January 6 after the New Year, aligning with their Mexica customs. As December's chill swept through their village each year, a group of white women—wives of the wealthy owners of the smelting company—would arrive. They came bearing gifts—boxes filled with food, clothes, and sometimes toys. Their appearance was striking too: well dressed, faces smiling, moving with a grace and ease that seemed unattainable. These women seemed to come from another world, one full of possibilities and comfort. After these visits, Abuela Tupina's grandmother would sit her down by the fire, her rough hands gently braiding her granddaughter's long dark hair.

"These people live on the other side, 'el otro lado,' where life is more comfortable," her grandmother would explain softly, her voice a mix of resignation and wonder.

Abuela Tupina's grandmother was a curandera. She practiced curanderismo, a traditional Latin American system of holistic healing that integrates natural remedies and cultural practices to address physical, emotional, and spiritual well-being.[4] She instilled in Abuela Tupina the importance of education as a path to a different world beyond their dusty village. These stories, interwoven with lessons on healing herbs, food as medicine, and spiritual rituals passed down through generations, ignited Abuela Tupina's curiosity and ambition.

At the age of six, Abuela Tupina relocated with her family to a modest community in Ciudad Juárez, right at the heart of the US–Mexico border. Though her family's home was in Mexico, Abuela Tupina had secured a coveted spot to attend private school in El Paso, Texas, beginning in middle school. This marked the beginning of a daily journey across a geographical, political, and cultural divide. Each morning, she would walk for miles along with a small group of cross-border students, their footsteps tracing the line between two worlds. School became the place where Abuela Tupina could weave the traditional healing arts she learned from her grandmother with the disciplines of Western medicine and science. Between her drive to learn and her deep-rooted desire to heal, she rose to the top of her class, where she graduated with honors and a college scholarship.

With a call to holistic healing, she earned a bachelor's degree in psychology and a master's degree in social work at the University of Texas. Throughout her academic and professional journey, Abuela Tupina stayed intimately connected to her heritage, dedicating herself to the study and instruction of Mexica holistic healing practices. As a mentor and an instructor, Abuela Tupina honored the lineage of curanderas before her, passing down much of her knowledge orally as her ancestors had done. For Abuela Tupina, these professional pursuits were also a reclamation and celebration of the ancient rituals and remedies that had nurtured and sustained her people long before European boots touched North American soil.

By the time COVID-19 struck, Abuela Tupina had built a respectable career and a family. But between December 2020 and January 2021, she faced unimaginable grief as four cherished members of her community succumbed to the virus.

"In Mexica culture," Abuela Tupina explained, "death isn't merely an end but a transition, a moment of transcendence. It's a journey from this life to the next, where spirits are guided by the love and rituals of their kin. COVID stripped us of these sacred traditions. We firmly believe that the only certainty in life is death. So, how one leaves this world matters profoundly to us."

For the Mexica and many other Indigenous communities, the transition from life to death traditionally unfolds through rituals and communal celebrations that honor the departed while reinforcing cultural heritage. These ceremonies also offer a space for storytelling and the transmission of wisdom, preserving cultural identity and continuity when a member departs.

The COVID-19 pandemic blocked time-honored passages to the other side due to the virus's sudden and isolating nature. While communities attempted to preserve cultural practices through virtual or electronic means, these attempts fell short of capturing the depth and significance of these ceremonies. As each person passed, particularly tribal elders, priceless cultural knowledge and history were lost, leaving permanent scars on the collective spirit of Indigenous communities across the nation and globe.

Determined to keep her traditions alive even in the face of such profound loss, Abuela Tupina began a daily ritual at home: setting up altars adorned with fresh flowers, lighting copal incense (a fragrant tree resin used for spiritual cleansing), and offering prayers to honor her loved ones and preserve their memory amid the erasure of life and culture.

The devastation of COVID on Indigenous communities was global. In the US, Native Americans and Alaska Natives were 2.6 times more likely to die from COVID-19 than white Americans.[5] In Canada, First Nations people experienced a COVID death rate that was 4.5 times higher than non-Indigenous peoples. In Australia, Indigenous communities were twice as likely to be infected,[6] and in New Zealand, Māori and Pacific communities were significantly more likely to be hospitalized.[7]

Like many in their community, Abuela Tupina's sister battled high blood pressure and diabetes—conditions disproportionately affecting Indigenous populations in the US. Along with obesity, asthma, and lung diseases, these chronic health issues affected their daily lives as well as increased their risk of severe complications and death from COVID-19.[8]

Diabetes is nearly three times more common among Native Americans and Alaska Natives than among non-Hispanic/Latino white adults,[9] with 16 percent of Indigenous Americans affected compared to 8.5 percent of non-Hispanic/Latino whites.[10] Obesity rates are also notably high in Native American communities, often exceeding those seen in Hispanic/Latino and Black populations.[11] Hypertension follows a similar trend, with Indigenous adults facing significantly higher risks than non-Hispanic/Latino whites.[12] Native Americans and Alaska Natives are also 20 percent more likely to suffer from asthma[13] and experience higher rates of cardiovascular disease and certain cancers, including liver, stomach, kidney, lung, colorectal, and breast cancer, than non-Hispanic/Latino white people.[14] Overall, Indigenous Americans have a life expectancy that is about 5.5 years shorter than the national average.[15]

To effectively address these disparities, it's essential to understand how they came to be. The notion that poor health among Indigenous communities is simply due to lifestyle choices or genetic predisposition[16] is both incomplete and misleading. The roots of Indigenous health disparities are shaped significantly by discriminatory policies and practices throughout history.[17] Their health reflects broader systemic problems, including past injustices, social and economic inequities, environmental damage, limited access to quality health care, and racism in medicine. Collectively, these factors exacerbate the risk and severity of health conditions among Indigenous peoples today.

In the sweltering heat of July 2014, I attended my first powwow with Luke, hosted by the Nipmuc Nation. I was pregnant with our first child at the time, and his aunts and cousins greeted me with excitement, eagerly welcoming the prospect of a new member joining their community. As I watched the vibrant celebrations unfold, I found myself wanting to learn more about their history, customs, and especially the foods that had sustained their community for generations. Later that day, I turned to Google, hoping to find some traditional recipes from the Nipmuc or other tribes native to Massachusetts to try and share with our growing family. Most of the search results, to my dismay, led me to fried dough recipes. My conversations with Luke's Native American family members often turned to recipes with heavy Western influence, like bread pudding. I knew that many Indigenous practices, including cooking, were passed down orally rather than readily categorized in cookbooks or websites. I also remembered from my history classes that Native American food traditions were far more varied and plant-based than what I was finding.

Ten years later, I had the unexpected joy of preparing and tasting fresh, Indigenous food, made from recipes that had been handed down over time. In October of 2024, I emailed Abuela Tupina, thanking her for the gift of sharing her time and her story with me. She replied, "[We have our] Moondance ceremony coming in November. If you feel called to come and experience ceremonial life for a week, let me know."

The Moondance Ceremony, known as *La Danza Huitzilmeztli* among the Mexica, is an ancient, weeklong spiritual and healing ritual practiced by Indigenous peoples of North and Mesoamerica. Held during the full moon in the fall, it honors the strength of women who give birth, fertility, the cycles of nature, the earth, and the ancestors. The ceremony weaves together dancing, fasting, prayer, and other sacred rituals like *temazcal* (a Nahuatl word meaning "house of heat" or sweat lodge) to foster physical, emotional, and spiritual healing. Moondancers fast for four days and nights, dancing and praying under the moonlight, while invited supporters like me assist by preparing food, providing childcare, tending the fire, working in the medicine tent, and providing encouragement to the Moondancers as they dance under the moonlight. No alcohol or substances are used during this time, except for ceremonial tobacco. Electronics are also set aside, as the ceremony takes place in harmony with nature—camping under the open sky, cooking from scratch outdoors, waking with the sunrise, and resting as night falls. It is a profound journey of community, resilience, and renewal that celebrates nature and the transformative power of women in nurturing and bringing forth life.

Camping is not my idea of fun (it's not even close to the top of my list), but this felt like an invitation I could not pass up. Without hesitation, I made plans for an impromptu trip to Manchaca, Texas, where Abuela Tupina hosts the annual La Danza. My good friend Lisa joined me from Boston to share in this experience. On arrival to the campgrounds, we were assigned to work in the kitchen, an essential role in the community, as we were tasked with feeding around sixty people each day. The outdoor kitchen, equipped with fresh running well water and grills, was led by Abuela Xochi, a woman with a stern face and a soft voice. A longtime friend of Abuela Tupina, she travels from Mexico every year to help her host La Danza and spoke only Spanish. I was grateful to find that the six years of Spanish I had taken came flooding back.

Abuela Xochi ran a tight kitchen. Under her expert guidance I, alongside a dozen supporters, prepared some of the freshest, tastiest meals I've ever had, using seasonal ingredients sourced from local farms. Each dish was a tribute to the culinary traditions passed down through generations of Mexica ancestors—ceviches made with juicy tomatoes, ripe avocados, crisp bell peppers, and citrus fruits; hearty soups made from carrots, potatoes, onions, and lentils; flavorful sides of black, pinto, and Mayan beans cooked with garlic and spices; pumpkin and sweet potato stews infused with the warm aromas of star anise and cinnamon; and vibrant salads that featured the most tender broccolini I've ever tasted. Whenever I remembered to put down my fork, I took notes, eagerly soaking in every detail so I could recreate these dishes at home and share them with my family.

About 90 percent of everything we made was plant-based, rooted in the earth and honoring the land. With only a small refrigerator, we couldn't store much meat, just as Indigenous peoples historically relied on minimal animal products. Elders and children were served first, with everyone encouraged to take only what they needed. Seconds were allowed only after each person had filled their plate. The food, along with the sense of community and the beauty of nature, nourished me in every way—mentally, physically, and spiritually. I felt more energized, balanced, and connected than I had in a long time.

Traditionally, Indigenous peoples in the Americas maintained diets rich in fruits, vegetables, whole grains, legumes, and proteins derived from foraging, agriculture, hunting, and fishing.[18] Their lifestyle, which involved considerable physical activity for survival and leisure, showed little evidence of chronic diseases like obesity, diabetes, or heart disease that are prevalent today. Alcohol was not routinely part of Indigenous life until European colonizers and explorers introduced this substance in large amounts to the Americas in the late fifteenth and sixteenth centuries.[19] Historical accounts also highlight an Indigenous population that experienced low incidence of chronic disease before European contact.[20]

The arrival of European colonizers marked the beginning of a seismic shift, introducing a slew of infectious diseases that were new and deadly to Indigenous communities. These included smallpox, bubonic plague, chicken pox, cholera, diphtheria, influenza, malaria, measles, scarlet fever, some sexually transmitted diseases, typhoid, typhus, tuberculosis, leptospirosis, and pertussis.[21] Smallpox was used as a deliberate biological weapon, notably with British forces distributing smallpox-infected blankets to tribes such as the Delawares and Shawnees from 1754 to 1763.[22] After European colonization, infectious diseases led to the deaths of up to 95 percent of Indigenous populations in the Americas, resulting in the loss of about twenty million people.[23]

Throughout the seventeenth and eighteenth centuries, European powers such as the British, French, and Spanish expanded their territories in the Americas, leading to increased conflict with and forced displacement of Indigenous populations. This set the stage for large-scale, systematic forced relocation. Perhaps the most well-known example from this period was the Indian Removal Act of 1830. This discriminatory policy forcibly relocated tribes east of the Mississippi River, including the Cherokee, Choctaw, Chickasaw, Creek, and Seminole, from their ancestral lands, pushing them further west and north, away from the land that colonizers were interested in occupying themselves.[24] This led to the Trail of Tears, a tragic journey during which about four thousand Cherokees perished over a grueling thousand-mile trek, resulting in profound and enduring impacts on their health and well-being.[25]

The designated "reservations" that Native Americans were forcibly relocated to were often characterized by poor agricultural potential and environmental degradation, exposing communities to pollutants and limiting access to sustainable food sources and clean water, air, and land.[26] These locations also isolated Indigenous communities from economic opportunities and perpetuated cycles of poverty that continue today.[27] Compounding these issues, the US government provided rations that were cheap, nonperishable, and nutritionally poor, such as lard, flour, sugar, and canned meat,[28] disrupting traditional diets and leading to long-term health issues like obesity, diabetes, and diet-related cancers.

Tribes experienced severe health declines as their cultural practices, community and family structure, and access to traditional food sources and clean environments were systematically shattered, leading to increased risk of disease and malnutrition. Health services on reservations were, and often still are, severely underfunded and understaffed, leaving many without access to adequate health care.[29] The Dawes Act of 1887 further undermined tribal cohesion by dividing communal lands into individual allotments, eroding economic stability, and increasing reliance on poor-quality government rations.[30]

This exploitation of people, land, and resources—driven by colonizers in the North and mining companies in the South—profoundly affected Abuela Tupina's ancestors and Indigenous communities across the continent. To date, Indigenous people have suffered centuries of forced relocation, often implemented through military action. Although the Indian Reorganization Act of 1934 aimed to counter some of the Dawes Act's effects by promoting tribal self-governance, it imposed Western-style governance structures on tribes.[31] The Termination Era of the 1950s sought to end federal recognition of tribes and dissolve tribal sovereignty, deepening political and legal marginalization and often making access to justice and health resources more complicated.[32] Collectively, these policies led to the dismantling of crucial health services, deepened poverty and social dislocation, and severely hindered tribes' ability to effectively address and advocate for their well-being based on their cultural and community needs.

At the heart of enduring health disparities in Indigenous communities lies the concept of *intergenerational trauma*—the transmission of trauma from one generation to the next.[33] Forced relocation, discriminatory policies in education, child welfare, and cultural assimilation inflicted lasting harm, particularly through family-child separation and cultural erasure.

Historically, the US and Canadian governments enacted policies to assimilate Indigenous peoples by removing children from their families and placing them in boarding schools or foster homes, where they were exposed to Western education, culture, and values.[34] These institutions subjected children to abuse, neglect, and harsh discipline, severing their connection to their heritage and, in some cases, leading to death.[35]

The forced removal of children was part of a broader effort to erase Indigenous cultures and languages, causing deep, intergenerational damage. In the mid-twentieth century, child-welfare policies disproportionately targeted Indigenous families, with social workers often using Euro-American standards to deem Indigenous parenting practices inadequate.[36] This contributed to long-term mental health challenges and a breakdown in community cohesion, as the trauma of family separation was passed down.

The effects of these traumatic experiences, systemically scaled through policy, continue to shape health today, even for descendants who did not directly experience the abuse. The lingering effects, including stress, anxiety, displacement, and erosion of family bonds, impact mental and physical health, social relationships, access to care and resources, and trust in institutions. A systematic review revealed that Indigenous adults in the US are at higher risk for post-traumatic stress disorder (PTSD), depression, suicide, and substance use disorder.[37] Suicide rates among Indigenous youth are also alarmingly high, two to three times than those of non-Indigenous youth.[38] Within health care, Indigenous women in the US and Canada were subjected to forced sterilizations as part of eugenics practices.[39] These practices, carried out without consent, deepened mistrust in the health care system.

This long-standing skepticism set the stage for the COVID-19 pandemic, which exacerbated existing physical health disparities as well as intensified intergenerational trauma and mental health challenges within Indigenous communities.[40] The abrupt loss of Indigenous elders, who serve as carriers of cultural knowledge, spiritual practices, and traditional teachings, devastated community cohesion and cultural resilience, particularly around ceremonial traditions such as Moondances, Sundances, powwows, and rituals around birth and death.[41]

Like many Indigenous leaders, Abuela Tupina had to pause La Danza during the early years of the pandemic. While the ceremony has since resumed, its cultural significance endures amid a painful history of systemic racism and intergenerational trauma.

Alongside the transmission of trauma, we can use the emerging field of *epigenetics* as a crucial perspective for understanding how these health disparities form. Epigenetics explores how environmental factors and life experiences can influence gene expression without changing the underlying

DNA sequence.[42] This field began to take shape in the early twentieth century, with British embryologist Conrad Waddington first introducing the term in 1942.[43] Through subsequent research, scientists discovered how environmental interactions can change the way our genes work, and how these changes can be passed down to future generations.[44]

Think of DNA as a blueprint for building and maintaining the body. Epigenetics adds another layer to this blueprint with "tags" or "markers" that determine which genes are turned on or off.[45] These markers can be influenced by factors like diet, stress, toxins, and social and environmental conditions. Over time, these influences can affect an individual's risk of chronic diseases, and the changes can be inherited by future generations.

Epigenetics sheds light on why health issues like diabetes, heart disease, and autoimmune conditions persist across generations in marginalized communities—even among those who adopt healthier behaviors, achieve higher socioeconomic status, or gain access to health care.[46] Poverty, historical trauma, ongoing discrimination, environmental stress, food insecurity, and inadequate health care create hostile living conditions that can alter epigenetic markers, influencing the expression of genes related to health and metabolism and increasing the risk of disease.[47] This framework highlights how Indigenous health disparities are deeply tied to historical and systemic factors that have shaped living conditions, access to resources, and genetic susceptibility across generations.

The cumulative impact of these disparities became glaringly apparent during COVID. Similar to low-income, Black, and Hispanic/Latino populations, Indigenous communities in the US faced disproportionate infection and mortality rates, far surpassing those in the broader population. A striking example is the Navajo Nation, which, at its peak, reported infection rates higher than some of the hardest-hit states, including New York and New Jersey.[48] The Navajo Nation, spanning Arizona, New Mexico, and Utah, became an epicenter of suffering and loss.

The pandemic's harsh effects were similarly felt by US Pacific Islanders, including the Marshallese community.[49] The Marshallese are an overlooked ethnic group in the conversation on racial health disparities because they are often grouped with the broader classification of Asian American and

Pacific Islander. The Marshallese people originate from the Republic of Marshall Islands, a vast chain of volcanic islands and atolls in the central Pacific Ocean. Known for their rich cultural history and deep-rooted family structure and community ties, the Marshallese have navigated life in the vast Pacific for centuries, sustaining themselves through fishing, agriculture, and the sharing of communal resources.

Like Indigenous Americans, the Marshallese have suffered a history of relocation, environmental devastation, and systemic marginalization. To develop and improve its nuclear arsenal during the Cold War era, the US conducted 67 nuclear tests on several of these islands from 1946 to 1958.[50] Among these tests was the Castle Bravo H-bomb dropped in 1954, which was 1,000 times the power of the Hiroshima bomb.[51] The extensive testing caused extreme environmental damage as well as immediate and long-term health and ecological impacts, forcing many Marshallese to leave their ancestral lands.[52]

The Compacts of Free Association, approved by the US Congress in 1986, permitted citizens from The Marshallese Islands and Micronesia visa-free entry to the US for work and education.[53] This policy provided an avenue for Pacific Islanders to escape the deteriorating conditions on their islands and seek opportunities abroad.[54]

Arkansas became a popular destination for the Marshallese due to job opportunities in the poultry industry, one of the largest agricultural products of the state.[55] Over time, a robust Marshallese community formed in Arkansas, supported by networks of family and friends that facilitated further migration. However, this concentration in low-income, high-density areas, coupled with limited access to health care, healthy food, and other essential services, left the Marshallese especially vulnerable to health disparities.

The significant challenges the Marshallese faced echoed the disruptions and disparities Native Americans endured. The nuclear testing and military actions drastically altered their native-built environment, leading to a reliance on high-fat, carbohydrate-rich foods like Spam and white rice—foods introduced through US aid—rather than their traditional diet of agricultural farming and fish.[56] Relocation to southern parts of the US introduced them to areas with poor healthy-food access, high fast-food density, limited walkability, and automobile dependence.

As a result, the Marshallese have disproportionately high rates of obesity and related chronic diseases today compared to other racial and ethnic populations both domestically and globally. My team's research, along with other studies on the Marshallese population in the US, reveals that obesity affects up to 61.7 percent of this community, while type 2 diabetes affects as many as 50 percent, rates that are more than four times higher than the national average for US adults.[57] And, despite comprising a small percentage of the US population, the Marshallese experienced a disproportionately high number of COVID-19 cases and deaths. This pattern repeated itself among Native Hawaiians, who also experienced environmental and lifestyle degradation and cultural erosion due to colonization, which contributed to disproportionately high rates of COVID-19 spread and fatalities.[58]

Historically, policies and initiatives aimed at addressing these disparities have fallen short. For Indigenous and Pacific Islander peoples, funding has been inconsistent and insufficient for essential services like health care, education, employment, and infrastructure. For example, the Indian Health Service (IHS), established to provide health care to Native Americans and Alaska Natives, has faced chronic underfunding. According to a 2022 US government report, the IHS received less than half of what was needed to meet its population's health care needs,[59] leading to limited access to medical services, outdated facilities, and insufficient staff, thus exacerbating health disparities.[60]

Effective public health requires acknowledging historical context and understanding the unique culture and needs of communities. Indigenous communities, each with its distinct language, culture, and traditions, are incredibly diverse. This means we must craft culturally relevant interventions that address shared experiences of systemic marginalization, respect unique cultural practices, and remove systemic barriers to health.

While I had read about culturally tailored interventions for Indigenous populations, it wasn't until I experienced La Danza firsthand that I began to understand what this looked like.

The Mexica practice holistic care, viewing health as an interconnected balance of physical, mental, emotional, and spiritual well-being. This perspective recognizes that individual health is interconnected with the health of the community and the environment. Indigenous peoples have long known that nature offers not just sustenance but profound healing properties. The concept of food as medicine reflects the belief that the land provides everything needed for well-being through plants, herbs, and the nourishing act of communal sharing. Together, these practices form a holistic approach to health, deeply intertwined with culture, spirituality, and a reverence for the earth.

At La Danza, I spoke with Felisa, a Moondancer, who shared insights about her midwifery work through the Luz de Atabey Midwifery Project as an example of culturally tailored care.[61] Through no-cost pop-up clinics, home visits, and telehealth, care centers the mother and is grounded in cultural traditions and collective values that honor the body, spirit, and community. It included providing food support for struggling families, offering assistance to keep mothers and their children in stable housing, and incorporating culturally rooted ceremonies that nurtured both body and spirit. Women preparing for birth were surrounded by songs, prayers, and traditional practices that honored the profound transformation of motherhood. After delivery, a six-week closing ceremony provided space for physical recovery and emotional healing, reinforcing each mother's vital role within her family and community.

The Mexica, along with many other Indigenous communities, also make it a point to acknowledge their past traumas head-on, embracing their heritage as a path to healing. This approach hit me deeply, especially since, in 2024, I had yet to fully confront the anti-Asian racism and the internalized self-loathing I had been trying to deny and escape. During La Danza, a group of supporters and I were invited to participate in a temazcal ceremony led by Abuela Xochi. This group ritual is a purification and therapeutic practice, using heat and steam to detoxify the body, relieve stress, and promote well-being.[62] It also serves as a spiritual practice, connecting participants to nature, their ancestors, and their community and facilitating emotional and mental healing from past traumas. Accompanied by prayer and chanting, the temazcal symbolizes the womb, offering a space for rebirth where old wounds are left behind and participants emerge spiritually renewed.

Remember when I said heat, humidity, and I don't get along? Well, we still don't (saunas are just a step above camping on my list of fun things to do), and I had half a mind to not get into the temazcal. But under the watchful eye of Abuela Xochi, and with an unyielding sense in my heart that I should at least try, I went in.

The temazcal was made from thick, unbreathable canvas. One by one, about twenty of us crawled in barefoot on our hands and knees, sitting cross-legged with our knees touching on a dirt floor. We filled the temazcal with two rows of circles. The only light came from a small opening, through which a firekeeper passed in heated stones. At the center, Abuela Xochi held a small pail, while Esme, a helper, used a ladle to pour water over the hot stones, releasing steam that increased the temperature inside with every passing second. The high humidity in a tightly enclosed space can make the heat in temazcals feel much more intense than regular saunas, with four rounds of prayers lasting up to two hours. Although I sat at the back, I could feel the cooler outside air from the opening of the temazcal. Then, the firekeeper closed the flap, plunging us into pitch-black darkness and rising heat.

"Is it supposed to be closed?" I asked an abuela beside me.

"Yes, we keep it closed."

Oh shit.

With sweat already dripping down my elbows, I reached down to feel the cool, reassuring earth beneath my fingers. Closing my eyes, I focused on my breath and the soothing cadence of Abuela Xochi's voice. She guided us through the first round of prayers, which on that day focused on childhood, family, and relationships. We honored lost childhood friends and mourned our own childhood experiences if we had to grow up too soon. Yet, the rising heat inside the temazcal made it difficult for me to focus. After the first round was complete, the entryway opened once more for the firekeeper to pass inside newly heated stones.

"If you are feeling unwell, this would be the time to leave," the abuela beside me advised. "However, once you leave, you cannot come back."

I slowly got up and made my way toward the opening.

"¿Qué pasa?" inquired Abuela Xochi.

"I feel faint," I said.

She firmly replied, "La medicina está funcionando. Vuelve a sentarte. Puedes sentarte junto a la abertura." (Translation: The medicine is working. Sit back down. You can sit by the opening.)

Feeling a mix of embarrassment and chagrin, I sat back down, grateful to be near the cooler entryway. From that point on, my mind was fully focused. Through group prayer, we were given space to reflect on parents or caregivers who may have fallen short of meeting our needs, while also celebrating the families we created when biological ones couldn't offer love and support. We embraced the practice of accepting ourselves—honoring our heritage, acknowledging our flaws, and celebrating our strengths—and we found healing in our cultural roots and native tongues. These prayers were interwoven with songs of both pain and joy, sung in Spanish and Nahuatl, which deepened the connection to our shared experiences. Tears flowed as we mourned personal losses and societal harm faced by families and nature around the world, while laughter echoed as we celebrated friendships, old and new, and the energy that comes from community and cultural pride.

I was struck by how easily light, joy, and humor emerged from a heavy topic in this shared space, even among strangers who had only met days before. In our affirmations, a central theme was duality, reflecting the natural world's contrasts: sun and moon, light and dark, cold and heat, life and death. We know pain because we have also known peace, we feel grief because we have experienced deep love. I discovered that the prayer prompts forced me to face memories and feelings I had buried—ones about my culture, heritage, and immigrant experience that were painful. In that small, sacred tent filled with community, I finally confronted these discomforts directly, processing them not as burdens to carry but as weights I could release.

Two hours later, we emerged from the tent, sweaty and muddy from the dirt that had mixed with our sweat, tears, and steam. We smiled, renewed in a way I hadn't expected. As each person stepped out, they were met with a deep embrace from the one who had gone before them. It was perhaps the most natural I have ever been—makeup-free, hair loosely gathered in a bun that had begun to unravel, sweaty, with traces of the earth on my face, arms, and legs, standing in the sunlight beneath a brilliant blue sky. We all looked that way. And the way we received each other was nothing short of a full acceptance of our truest, most vulnerable selves. In that moment, the discomfort I'd carried at times—unable to look at myself in the mirror—evaporated along with layers of societal pressures. It was a physical, emotional, and spiritual cleansing, a transformative experience that healed me in ways I could never find in a scientific article or a clinical setting.

La Danza deepened my appreciation for the power of cultural practices, which may not fit into the rigid, "evidence-based" Western frameworks of science but offer healing nonetheless. To address both the immediate health concerns and the deeper root causes of Indigenous health disparities, we must advocate a combined approach, blending downstream and upstream strategies with a holistic perspective on care.

It's vital to incorporate community and cultural expertise to design materials and services that are relevant to and resonate with different cultural populations. For example, the University of Saskatchewan's "Strong Bodies, Spirits, Minds, and Voices" initiative works closely with Indigenous communities to prevent type 2 diabetes among youth.[63] Through collaboration with elders, knowledge keepers, youth, and families, this initiative integrates Indigenous knowledge into the development of a culturally relevant health promotion toolkit. It combines traditional practices like healing circles, food as medicine, storytelling, and traditional dance with modern medical care, addressing both physical and cultural health needs, and demonstrating a holistic model for intervention. Similarly, the Navajo Nation's Diabetes Prevention Program incorporates traditional Navajo practices, such as farming and foraging for native foods, alongside teachings about a balanced diet rooted in their cultural heritage. By prioritizing community involvement, the program has improved participation and health outcomes, creating a sustainable model for health improvement.[64]

Centering communities is crucial for all marginalized groups facing health disparities.[65] The Partnership for Native American Cancer Prevention (NACP) demonstrates the power of community-centered solutions.[66] In collaboration with Northern Arizona University and the University of Arizona Cancer Center, NACP addresses the disproportionate cancer burden among Native Americans in the Southwest. The initiative emphasizes research, training, and outreach, all developed in partnership with Indigenous communities to improve cancer prevention and care. By integrating community involvement along the spectrum—from engagement to co-creation to empowerment[67]—researchers, policymakers, and health care providers can develop more equitable and effective health solutions.

Finally, as with all communities facing poor health, it's crucial to enact upstream policies and programs that target social and structural determinants. The Alaska Native Tribal Health Consortium (ANTHC) provides a comprehensive range of health care services to Alaska Natives and Native Americans across the state.[68] Through initiatives like traditional foods programs and expanded telehealth services, ANTHC improves access to specialized care for remote communities while also addressing immediate health needs and building sustainable health practices. Additionally, ANTHC's environmental health projects focus on mitigating the impact of environmental factors on physical and mental health, including ensuring access to clean water and preserving traditional food sources. By working to prevent exposure to contaminants and pollutants, ANTHC safeguards vital resources such as fish and game that are vital to the community's cultural and nutritional needs.

These examples show how blending traditional knowledge with modern health care and practicing health as a holistic balance of physical, mental, spiritual, and community well-being—as Abuela Tupina continues to do—can make a difference.

There's still much more to be done. We cannot go back and change the beginning. But we can start where we are now and change the ending.

CHAPTER 8

Do You See Me?

It was fall of 2016, and the crisp New England autumn air had already settled in. I lay sprawled down on our kitchen floor, feeling as though my responsibilities were pressing down on my lungs like an invisible weight. Hot tears trickled down my cheeks and onto the cool ceramic tiles, mixing with the faint scent of cinnamon oatmeal that Ivy, then nearly two years old, had spilled on the floor that morning.

Moments ago, I had dropped Ivy off at day care, a small parenting victory that involved navigating clothes wrestling, toothbrushing negotiations, breakfast coaxing, and a mini tantrum (hers, though I felt like throwing one myself). By the time I waved goodbye, I felt exhausted, even before my workday had begun. I was also in my second trimester with our second child, which seemed to make every ounce of stress I felt even heavier.

As I walked back into our house to prepare for a conference call, I was greeted with the chaotic aftermath of our exuberant rescue dog's latest episode of anxiety. Leo, our fifty-five-pound black-and-white tuxedo lab–pit-bull mix, was all muscle and energy, loving us with a fierce intensity that matched his fear of abandonment. He had once again channeled his distress at being left alone into a destructive outburst, this time targeting a doorframe. The damage was extensive—the wooden frame gouged and splintered, the mess sprawling across the floor.

"Leo!" I chided wearily.

He wagged his tail sheepishly, at peace now that I was home, and followed me dutifully to the kitchen. My mind had been set for me to get a broom and vacuum to tackle the mess, but my body had other plans. I found myself lying on the floor, where I took a few reluctant moments to cry.

At the time, Luke was in his third year of medical residency, his grueling twelve-plus hour shifts stretching into the late hours of the night and into the weekends. Personal, sick, and family leave time were virtually nonexistent for residents, particularly for new fathers. We planned for him to use all of his two weeks' vacation time to correspond with when Jade was due, as his residency program did not offer paid paternity leave. This arrangement, combined with the exhausting and unrelenting demands of residency, left him with little flexibility in his schedule and no semblance of work-life balance. As a result, I took on the role of primary caregiver of our growing family. It fell to me—yet again—to clean up the destruction, devise a new plan for Leo, and somehow squeeze these unexpected tasks into an already overflowing schedule.

As I knelt down to pick up the larger pieces of splintered wood, my growing belly pressing against my legs, a fresh wave of fatigue, frustration, and helplessness washed over me. My mental and physical energy were consumed by what felt like an unending list of personal responsibilities on top of substantial professional commitments.

As an expectant mom with a toddler, I maneuvered the cycle of diaper changes, bedtime stories, potty training, and soothing nightmares while dealing with the physical and emotional strains of pregnancy. As a wife, I offered emotional support while taking on the lioness's share of practical household responsibilities. The tasks felt endless, like a high-stakes one-woman circus. I balanced being the dog walker and trainer, the household cook, cleaner, grocery runner, laundry folder, chauffeur, appointment scheduler, event planner, and financial manager. Plus, I was the Emergency Snack Distributor, Finder of Lost Things, Chief Hair Stylist/Detangler (which positioned me well for the future role of Lice Remover), and Professional Toy Organizer, with a PhD in How to Trip Over Legos Without Losing Your Cool.

Many aspects of parenting I truly cherish, like making artwork together, seeing them get excited about our family traditions, like making fried spring rolls filled with leftovers the day after Thanksgiving, and laughing as they make up their own jokes and dance routines. And, many of the mundane aspects of parenting I do not enjoy.

On top of it all, I tried to maintain connections with important people in our lives as a friend, sister, and daughter. There was so much to juggle and new tricks to constantly learn, all while maintaining the illusion of control. Each hat I wore involved its own blend of physical and emotional labor, where much of the work was hidden from view but essential to keeping the show running.

This ongoing, invisible effort was compounded by my more visible professional commitments. As a full-time professor at Boston University and an adjunct professor at Harvard, I earned a higher salary than Luke as a resident. My role as the primary breadwinner at the time meant that my income was crucial to our family's financial stability and future. I'm deeply grateful to be passionate about my chosen line of work in public health, striving to excel and make a meaningful impact through research, teaching, and service. However, balancing rigorous professional demands with the constant, behind-the-scenes responsibilities of family life was a continual challenge, one that often left me feeling depleted.

Above all, I struggled with a heavy sense of guilt for feeling over-whelmed. I had a stable and fulfilling job that came with flexibility, autonomy, and competitive pay and benefits—advantages many would envy. As an academic, I had freedom to set my own schedule and create a work environment that suited me. We lived comfortably, benefiting from relatively high socioeconomic status, excellent health insurance, and access to quality health care. Our neighborhood offered abundant healthy food options, walking, biking, and hiking paths, and we were supported by a strong network of family, friends, and community. My mother provided part-time childcare for Ivy and would later do the same for Jade. This critical support allowed Luke and me to save more for a down payment on a house rather than paying the astronomical price of full-time childcare in the Boston area. Even with part-time help, childcare still consumed roughly 25 percent of our disposable income at the time.

Given these advantages, it seemed like our set of social determinants should position us for a good quality of life. Yet, I couldn't shake the feeling that I was failing to manage everything as well as I should. I had accepted that working and parenting would be challenging (or at least I thought I had), but wasn't I supposed to be adapting and getting better as a working mom? *What was wrong with me?*

The guilt was a constant shadow that questioned my right to feel stressed and overwhelmed. The awareness of my advantages clashed with my feelings of inadequacy, creating a constant, internal friction. Though outwardly the surface seemed smooth, internally I felt like I was flailing and failing to be everything I loved and aspired to be: a public health professional, a mom, a wife, a daughter, a friend, a runner, an artist, a baker. The physical and mental requirements of growing my career while growing my family was stretching me to my limits.

Despite being surrounded by family and friends, I felt an acute sense of isolation. However, I know I was not alone in feeling lonely. My experience is part of a broader phenomenon affecting many women, caregivers, and other marginalized groups, who frequently shoulder the dual burden of meeting professional demands while managing extensive personal responsibilities.

It would be tempting to frame my work-life experience as more difficult than Luke's. But my story is intertwined with his, our struggles different but connected in their impact on our family dynamics. As professionals in academia and medicine, we each faced unique obstacles: I grappled with balancing academic responsibilities and managing a heavier share of household and parenting duties, while Luke contended with the relentless physical and psychological demands and inflexibility of his job as a doctor.

Luke's years as a resident physician were consumed by long hours at the hospital with brief, irregular breaks. The demands of medical training and providing care were intense, marked by the constant need to make high-stakes decisions, manage a large caseload, and perform a myriad of medical tasks under significant pressure. This rigidity and the lack of flexibility meant that Luke had scant time for sleep, fitness, personal activities, friends, or family life, contributing to significant stress and fatigue.

Even though it did not always feel like Luke was contributing equitably, the reality was that what constituted full effort for each of us was quantitatively and qualitatively distinct. This difference in work-life capacity was largely shaped by the demands of our respective jobs (my job's flexibility in direct contrast with his job's rigidity), as well as by societal norms and traditional gender roles that mold expectations of responsibilities. It took me several years of navigating marriage, work, and parenting to begin to grasp this complexity. And we are still learning, making mistakes, and making adjustments.

Acknowledging both of our realities requires us to understand the structural factors and work stressors that shape the complexity of work-life balance. Our story is one of many that illustrates how struggles in one domain often ripple through every aspect of life, affecting not just individuals but families, communities, and populations as a whole. This chapter is about confronting the realities of job stress, undervalued and unseen labor, and the mental and physical toll it takes on those who bear it. By exploring these challenges, we can also uncover pathways to do better.

The average full-time worker dedicates one-third of their waking hours to their job.[1] With so much of our lifetime devoted to work, our physical and mental well-being is significantly impacted by the way work is designed, known as *job design*. Robert Karasek, a renowned psychologist and occupational health expert, pioneered a framework to explore how different aspects of job design affect our well-being. His 1979 Job Demands-Control Model was developed from extensive research, including national surveys in Sweden and the United States.[2]

Imagine the model as a simple grid with four squares, or quadrants. These quadrants are divided by two axes, each ranging from high to low. On one axis, we have *job demands*, which reflect how much work we have, how challenging it is, and the physical and psychological pressures a job requires. On the other axis, we have *job control*, which reflects how much influence and autonomy we have over our own work, such as how to do our tasks and the ability to set our own pace and schedule. Combining these two dimensions creates four quadrants:

High Strain Quadrant—High Demands, Low Control: This is often the most stressful work situation because the workload is heavy, mentally or physically demanding, and workers have little say in how to manage it. Example professions: firefighters, policemen, emergency health care providers, restaurant service staff.

Active Quadrant—High Demands, High Control: Workers have high work demands as well as some power to make decisions about how to handle it, which can help reduce stress. Example professions: managers, physicians, public officials.

Passive Quadrant—Low Demands, Low Control: Work demands are relatively lighter compared to other professions, but workers do not have much control over how things are done. This can be less stressful but may feel unsatisfying. Example professions: customer support representatives, data entry personnel, cleaning staff, delivery personnel, security personnel.

Low Strain Quadrant—Low Demands, High Control: Workers experience relatively low psychological demands and a good deal of control over their tasks, in which Karasek deemed the least stressful and most fulfilling situation. Example professions: freelance consultants, research scientists, engineers, architects.

Each quadrant helps us understand how stress and health are affected by different job aspects such as workload, pace, task variety, and autonomy.[3] Research on Karasek's model reveals that working in high-stress environments with heavy demands and minimal control is harmful to health.[4] Studies including meta-analyses indicate that workers in these high-strain roles are more prone to developing cardiovascular diseases, along with mental health issues like anxiety and depression, and experience overall physical decline.[5] In contrast, jobs that offer greater control and autonomy are associated with higher job satisfaction, lower stress levels, and better mental and physical health.[6]

While Karasek's model provides a useful foundation, it does not capture the distinct work experiences and stressors faced by different demographic groups. The model also overlooks the additional physical and emotional challenges associated with working through pregnancy, childbirth, postpartum care, and long-term caregiving responsibilities. To address these complexities, we must understand the balance between job demands and control in the context of other social and structural determinants. By considering these broader influences, we can better understand and address job stress through a more comprehensive approach to workplace well-being.

Though often used interchangeably, job stress and burnout represent different aspects of workplace well-being, with distinct implications. *Job stress* typically arises from everyday pressures and demands at work, which can often be managed with appropriate strategies or changes in workload. In contrast, *burnout* is a deeper, more persistent state of exhaustion and disconnection that requires focused interventions.[7] Defined by the 11th Revision of the International Classification of Diseases as an occupational phenomenon rather than a medical condition, burnout stems from chronic, unmanaged workplace stress. It is marked by deep energy depletion, a sense of cynicism or detachment from one's job, and a significant decline in professional effectiveness.[8]

Burnout rates have surged across professions and countries in recent years. In the US, burnout is highest among workers in health care (50–84 percent),[9] social work (62 percent),[10] and education (44–40 percent),[11] driven by high workloads, intense job demands, inadequate support, and limited control over their work environment. A 2023 survey of over 10,000 global workers found that 42 percent of workers reported experiencing burnout, the highest level recorded since May 2021.[12] These figures reflect broader changes in job demands and workplace conditions, emphasizing the urgent need to develop effective strategies to support worker well-being and prevent severe, long-term health issues.

This need is especially crucial for marginalized groups, who often face compounded challenges in the workplace due to systemic inequities that intersect, especially heightened job stress, burnout, and poor health.[13] For example, individuals from lower socioeconomic backgrounds often face fewer opportunities and significant barriers to securing stable, well-paying jobs with benefits,[14] contributing to heightened stress and burnout, along with limited ability to protect their health. Employees of color encounter barriers to equal pay, career advancement, and access to professional opportunities and are more likely to have lower-paying or less secure jobs.[15] Women, especially those of color, face pay gaps, limited advancement opportunities, and higher expectations for balancing work and domestic responsibilities.[16] This combination of factors exacerbates stress and impacts overall job satisfaction and health.

Such challenges are deeply intertwined with the evolving job landscape. This is particularly evident today in the rise of nonstandard work arrangements, such as subcontracted, temporary, on-call, and freelance positions. According to the Bureau of Labor Statistics, about 15.5 million US workers, or roughly 1 in 10, were in such roles in 2017, whereas other sources put the estimate closer to 1 in 3.[17] These nonstandard positions typically offer lower pay, minimal job security, inadequate protections, and fewer benefits, making working life even more difficult for marginalized workers.

Temporary help-agency roles, which numbered 2.2 to 2.7 million in 2024,[18] have grown four times faster than overall US employment since the end of the Great Recession. These roles often come with greater work hazards, particularly in high-risk industries like construction and manufacturing. Research shows that temporary workers are twice as likely to be injured on the job than full-time employees.[19] Women and people of color are disproportionately represented in these precarious jobs, with 25.9 percent of temporary positions occupied by Black workers and 25.4 percent by Hispanic/Latino workers, despite these groups' smaller overall proportions in the workforce.[20]

The overrepresentation of marginalized groups in temporary jobs underscores inequities in occupational distribution, as well as highlights the larger issue of job insecurity and its impact on health. The constant fear of losing one's job creates chronic stress that exacerbates physical and mental health issues,[21] particularly when compounded by unpredictable work schedules common among temporary, gig, and shift workers. Lack of job stability also limits access to vital resources like health benefits and mental health services. Research reveals that workers of color, low socio-economic workers, and immigrants face more job insecurity compared to their white, higher socioeconomic, and nonimmigrant counterparts.[22]

Job insecurity is linked to several health issues and poor health behaviors.[23] An analysis of a national sample of 17,000 American workers found that those with job insecurity have nearly five times the risk of serious mental illness and are more prone to pain conditions and chronic diseases like diabetes and heart disease.[24] These workers are also more likely to sleep poorly, smoke daily, miss work, have obesity, and experience worsening health. The same study also found gender differences: women facing job insecurity reported higher rates of asthma, diabetes, and work-life imbalance, while men reported higher rates of work absenteeism, chest pain, and hypertension.

Conversely, job security improves job satisfaction[25] and reduces work-related stress, leading to fewer sick days and increased productivity and collaboration.[26] A study from England found that companies providing job-sharing or enhanced job security saw up to six fewer days of absenteeism per employee each year.[27] Our team's study of a nationally representative sample of over 18,000 working US adults showed that job security is crucial for mental health, with having a secure job linked to a 25 percent reduction in severe psychological distress.[28]

Our research also showed that job flexibility, such as the ability to set one's own schedule, work from home, or take time off, can significantly improve mental health, reducing the likelihood of severe psychological distress by 26 percent. Flexible work arrangements help employees balance work and personal responsibilities, reducing stress and enhancing overall well-being. By allowing adjustments in work hours or location, employees can more effectively manage competing demands, including accessing health care,[29] leading to improved overall health in the long term. Another study of ours also revealed that women with low job flexibility worked more days while sick than men in similar roles, underscoring how limited autonomy can disproportionately burden women and compromise their ability to take care of their health.[30] Having job flexibility is particularly important given the "double shift" phenomenon, where working women manage both paid employment and extensive unpaid domestic work.[31]

Research highlights the sheer significance of this imbalance. According to the 2023 American Time Use Survey, working women spent about 2.4 hours per day on housework and childcare, while working men spent 1.6 hours daily.[32] This translates to working women spending about 50 percent more time on home and family responsibilities compared to their male counterparts. Although there has been some progress since the 1960s, the gender imbalance in the division of domestic responsibilities continues despite female contributions to the workforce.

This gendered double shift takes a serious toll on women's health.[33] Regardless of marital status, working women spend significantly more time on housework than men. This disparity is most pronounced in heterosexual marriages, where married women pre-COVID dedicated about 40 hours per week to domestic tasks compared to 16 hours per week among married men.[34] Working women who take on more than half the household responsibilities report higher stress levels, increased fatigue, and greater depression, anxiety, and psychological distress compared to men.[35] The double shift isn't just a concept—it's a lived experience for many women that profoundly impacts their well-being.

On a cloudy morning in early March of 2020, the news hit me like a cold wave. Ivy and Jade's day care was closing for two weeks, in sync with the public school closures due to the arrival of COVID-19. At the time, Ivy was five and scheduled to start kindergarten in the fall, and Jade was about to turn three. As a primary care physician and first responder, Luke returned to his long hours at work, donning his COVID protection gear early each morning and returning late in the evenings. He, alongside other health care providers, took on unprecedented personal and professional challenges in high-risk environments. At home, I faced a different set of challenges.

"Okay," I told myself, "two weeks. I can handle two weeks at home. It's just a short burst. I'll manage to stay on top of my projects while looking after the kids."

With a hopeful resolve, I dove into making adjustments like a seasoned acrobat to balance work and childcare. After all, I'd weathered other storms before, and I was confident I could navigate this one. I created a "learning corner" for Ivy and Jade with a colorful array of educational toys, books, and art supplies to keep them engaged. My master plan included alternating between Zoom meetings, mealtime, emails, child educational activities, my research and writing, supervised play and outdoor time, and PBS Kids—a well-orchestrated circus act that existed only in my mind. This grand vision lasted about a day before reality reminded me that no schedule survives first contact with a toddler and a prekindergartner.

Then came the dreaded extension: day care would remain closed for six weeks, aligning with the public school closures. What had begun as a short-term disruption was now morphing into an endurance test. My initial optimism quickly dissolved into mounting anxiety as I faced the daunting reality of juggling my full-time research, writing, and teaching responsibilities at home. With Luke at work, no partner to share the load, and no childcare centers or schools open, the situation was starkly different from when I was on maternity leave. It wasn't so much "working from home" as "parenting while working."

Still, I tried to reassure myself: *Six weeks is not forever. There's still an end in sight.*

But as the weeks passed, the situation grew bleaker. The announcement came: day care would be closed through the end of the school year; it was unknown if camps would be open for the summer. The walls of my home seemed to close in as I processed the news.

I'm screwed. That familiar sinking, suffocating feeling—the weight of invisible labor pressing on my lungs—came back.

The reality of having two young children at home for several more months, without the reprieve of childcare, school, or any extended family or neighbors to help, was too much to ask of working families. And yet, governments, workplaces, and schools had made it clear: this was the new norm, one in which parents, children, teachers, and employees all suffered.

As I looked around at the toys scattered across the floor, a new wave of exhaustion washed over me. The lines between work and home had blurred into a messy blend of Zoom meetings, virtual teaching, writing, endless requests for snacks, and preparing and cleaning up after three meals a day. In the chaos, I returned to the childhood routines that had brought me structure, crafting a schedule much like the ones my dad used to create for me. This time, however, my schedule was heavily reliant on screen time. I also turned once more to my mom for help. Though she worked full-time as a nurse's aide in a nursing home and was stretched thin, she managed to carve out two days during the week to help with childcare from April to June of that year.

When the girls were home with me, we started the day with breakfast, followed by two hours of PBS Kids for them while I tackled meetings and emails. Next came outdoor play (weather permitting) and lunch for all three of us, then some semi-independent playtime before the kids got another dose of PBS Kids. Dinnertime was followed by bath time. Rinse and repeat. With two young children constantly on the move, carving out time for focused work during the day was often impossible. I became a nocturnal worker, squeezing in my research and writing from 9 p.m. to midnight after the kids were finally asleep. On weekends, when Luke was around, I'd grab a few extra hours to write. This schedule became my daily survival guide that also quickly proved to be unsustainable.

As I juggled the demands of work and parenting during the first years of COVID, the reality of the double shift became even more pronounced. My personal struggle was a microcosm of a global social crisis. The COVID-19 pandemic thrust millions of women into the deep end of unpaid domestic, schooling, and childcare responsibilities.[36] Lockdowns, which abruptly removed the already shrinking "village" of support for modern women, and the shift to remote work, greatly intensified the burden, adding billions of hours of unpaid female labor globally.[37] Women and caregivers everywhere found themselves managing a tidal wave of professional and personal demands without the usual support systems.

The impact of the intensified double shift during the COVID-19 pandemic on health was substantial. A study of caregivers of five- to eighteen-year-old children in the US, UK, Canada, and Australia found that women shouldered disproportionately higher caregiving responsibilities than men during the pandemic, which was linked to elevated levels of distress and anxiety.[38] Another study of over 11,000 US mothers found that those experiencing significant pandemic hardships, such as disruptions due to balancing remote work and childcare, had greater levels of traumatic stress.[39] Though the immediate health dangers of COVID have subsided, the social, economic, and health ripple effects of the pandemic have not. Women across the globe continue to report spending more time on domestic work now than before 2020,[40] and nearly 2 million women in the US alone dropped out of the workforce entirely during COVID.[41] Given these challenges, what can we do to protect workers, families, and communities when the next crisis strikes?

To develop effective and equitable strategies, it's crucial to understand the historical context that has shaped our current society. Labor policies have traditionally reflected and reinforced societal norms rather than challenging them. For example, the long-standing view of men as primary breadwinners and women as primary caregivers,[42] combined with male-dominated boards and executive teams across professions,[43] has deeply influenced labor policy development and job design. Consequently, labor laws and norms often prioritize the needs of men in full-time roles.[44]

At the dawn of the twentieth century, labor policies focused on improving basic worker protections, addressing hazardous conditions, securing fair wages, and regulating working hours.[45] These measures aimed to safeguard male industrial workers in the manufacturing sector but often neglected the needs of women, people of color, and those in nontraditional roles.[46] This meant that many workers lacked essential protections, which set the stage for occupational health disparities.

Significant advancements like the Fair Labor Standards Act of 1938 established minimum wage and maximum working hours.[47] Yet, these improvements did not reach everyone equally. Domestic workers and agricultural laborers—many of whom were women and people of color—were frequently excluded from these protections.[48] This exclusion perpetuated health inequities, as those in lower-wage, less secure jobs often faced greater physical and mental health risks and fewer benefits such as sick leave and health insurance.

During World Wars I and II, millions of women entered the workforce in unprecedented numbers to fill roles vacated by men who went to fight.[49] Many of these women remained in the workforce after World War II, driven in part by the need for additional economic stability and newfound opportunities for financial independence.[50] Western countries including the US experienced economic growth post–World War II, which raised the standard of living for the middle class and catalyzed consumerism. This shift further shaped social expectations, making it both more common and financially advantageous for women to remain in the workforce.[51]

As more women entered and remained in the workforce, the inadequacies of existing labor policies became starkly apparent. These policies largely left unaddressed wage discrimination, limited opportunities, and insufficient protection for women and workers of color,[52] while inadequate paid parental leave and support worsened stress and health for working parents and children.[53] This historical neglect has led to intersecting occupational, gender, racial, and socioeconomic health inequities that prevail today.

In recent decades, US policymakers have made notable strides toward more health-promoting labor policies. For instance, the Family and

Medical Leave Act (FMLA) of 1993 marked a significant step forward by providing job-protected leave for new parents and individuals dealing with serious health conditions.[54] Efforts to achieve equal pay have shrunk the US gender wage gap, though it is still larger for older women and varies by race and ethnicity.[55]

Still, the US remains one of the few developed countries without a paid parental-leave policy. Research consistently shows that countries with paid parental leave have better outcomes in child health and development, parental health, family well-being, and population health.[56] While the average duration of paid maternity leave in OECD countries is around 18 weeks, the range is wide—from 43 weeks in Greece to none in the US, though some states offer paid leave.[57] Paid leave for fathers is much shorter or nonexistent, averaging 2.3 weeks in OECD countries. To address these disparities, labor policies must be strengthened to better support work-life balance for all parents and caregivers, with a particular focus on addressing gaps in countries like the US.

We can learn valuable lessons from countries with comprehensive parental leave and gender equality policies. For instance, Sweden offers up to 480 days (16 months) of paid leave per child[58] while Norway provides 49 weeks.[59] Both countries' policies encourage parents across genders to take time off and share child-rearing responsibilities. Nations like Finland and Iceland also support shared parenting with up to 160 working days of parental leave per parent[60] and 6 months of paid leave per parent, respectively.[61] In Iceland, parents who experience miscarriage after 18 weeks of pregnancy or a stillbirth after 22 weeks of pregnancy have the right to parental leave—a policy that does not yet exist in the United States. By adopting similar policies, nations like the US could significantly ease the burden on working parents, promote shared child-rearing responsibilities, and set new standards for valuing working families.

In August 2024, the US surgeon general issued a report on the severe challenges of parenting, noting that nearly half of parents struggle with intense stress, loneliness, and financial worries that contribute to worsening mental and physical health.[62] This official recognition stresses the need for systemic support to help parents manage their responsibilities, reduce their stress, and improve their own and their family's well-being.

This historical and global context underscores the current reality and possibilities of advocating for policies and practices that better support the needs of all workers and drive meaningful reform. Achieving fair pay is a crucial step toward a supportive and healthier workforce. This requires comprehensive strategies, including transparent pay practices, regular pay audits and revisions, ensuring fair pay during hiring, and clear compensation policies.[63]

Flexible work arrangements are increasingly vital, especially for working parents, caregivers, and those with disabilities. To promote flexibility, organizations can implement policies that allow for adjustable work hours, provide resources for hybrid and remote collaboration, and offer training for managers on effectively supporting workers in these arrangements.[64] Additionally, organizations should consider long-term strategies such as flexible employee contracts and career development opportunities to enhance job security and promote skill growth.[65]

Providing fair career advancement opportunities is essential for the health of organizations and their workforce. Companies can focus on reforming organizational policies and practices, such as adopting inclusive interview and hiring processes, reviewing and updating job descriptions and qualifications to eliminate biases, implementing transparent promotion criteria, providing training for managers, and establishing robust mentorship and sponsorship programs to support career advancement for eligible workers that may be overlooked for executive, managerial, or advancement opportunities.[66]

Providing affordable childcare is also critical to lessen the "double shift" burden and encourage women to participate in the workforce. The high cost of childcare in the US consumes an average of 24 percent of a household's income (up to 39 percent for low-income households), creating financial strain and impacting job performance, satisfaction, and retention.[67] By offering subsidized childcare and expanding the child tax credit, employers and policymakers can better support employees in managing both their professional and family responsibilities and improving the health of employees and their families.[68]

Comprehensive paid parental, medical, and sick leave is necessary to support employees during times of health issues or family responsibilities.

In addition to the lack of guaranteed parental leave, the US also lacks a federal mandate for paid sick leave.[69] A robust paid leave policy allows employees to take necessary time off without the fear of losing income, leading to better health and enhanced workplace productivity and retention. By investing in these key areas of reform, organizations can create more inclusive and supportive work environments that significantly enhance the health of employees, families, and communities.

The question, "what is wrong with me?" still crosses my mind from time to time, but less frequently now that I've gained a bit more wisdom and experience, the girls have grown more independent, Luke's work offers more flexibility and autonomy, and I've let go of the weight of a few expectations. It became clearer that we weren't meant to do it all alone after I returned home from La Danza, where everyone had one primary role in the community—cooking, childcare, healing, cleaning, firekeeping, or moondancing. No one person was expected to shoulder all responsibilities of daily living; we leaned on each other, which cultivated balance, structure, deep appreciation, social connection, and respect.

Instead of expecting working women and caregivers to have superpowers and be safety nets, juggling everything flawlessly in a world not designed for them, we can build better support systems to catch them and help them land on their feet. This chapter is for all who continue to wrestle with work-life challenges and those who can do something about it; for Leo, who perhaps saw me most fully during my struggles and loved me wholeheartedly through them; and for my mom, who still catches me when I stumble and cheers me on when I soar.

CHAPTER 9

The Light in the Dark

B ack in Panola, Alabama, the rising sun cast a warm glow over the town, illuminating the modest homes with wide porches sprinkled through the vibrant greens of the surrounding countryside. Inside Dorothy's unassuming general store, the shelves lay stocked with essentials: cans of chicken noodle soup, creamed corn, beans, and jars of dill pickles. Bottled water and brightly colored sodas sat next to boxes of pasta and packets of ramen, while over-the-counter fever and cough medicine awaited customers in need. And right up front at the checkout was a CDC infographic about COVID precautions.

"Even though we're a small town, COVID changed us too," Dorothy said. "So many lost a mother, a father, a sister, a brother."*

In early 2021, the COVID-19 vaccine became available in the US, but the nearest vaccination site to Panola was nearly forty miles away. This left the community largely unvaccinated and without any scheduled mobile clinics to provide access. Determined to change this, Dorothy called hospital after hospital, only to discover that Panola needed a minimum of forty names and signatures to secure a mobile vaccine clinic.

"I woke up every day thinking, 'How can we do it? How can we get the vaccine to Panola?' And something came to me: you need to do it," she said, her voice steady and serious.

---

*This chapter is informed by both a personal interview with Dorothy Oliver on May 5, 2022, and her appearance in the documentary, *The Panola Project*, directed by Jeremy Levine and Rachael DeCruz in 2021.

Dorothy reached out to her longtime friend and colleague, Commissioner Drucilla Russ-Jackson. With four decades of friendship and trust between them, Dorothy knew Drucilla was the kind of leader and community advocate who could step up to help.

To gather the forty names needed, Dorothy knew she had to reach out to her neighbors directly. With many lacking internet access, in-person conversations and phone calls were the primary means of communication. Her store, a tiny one-story building, became a hub of information and support. Whenever business was slow, she picked up her cell phone, her Alabama drawl calm and soothing as she reached out to fellow residents.

"Hey, Janelle, this is Dorothy," she began, her voice warm and familiar.

"Hey, Tim, how ya doin'? Do you need my help?"

"We're trying to bring the vaccine to Panola. If you see someone who hasn't been vaccinated, refer them to me, ya hear?"

"Hey, Janet! I was callin' to check if you got your COVID shot?"

Each call was a connection in a time of isolation and fear. Her conversations revealed the skepticism that lingered in the community. Many were hesitant, wary of the vaccine's safety. While the older residents were more open to discussing the vaccine, many younger people worried about the potential side effects or risks to their own health or their families.

"You keep me informed," a neighbor replied, uncertainty coming through in his voice as he hesitated to add his name to the list—a feeling that resonated throughout many homes in Panola.

"They give me all kind of reasons, so I just continue to encourage them," Dorothy said. "People don't know much about the vaccine—where to get it, what to expect, they really don't. It's important to talk to them and just give them some information."

The emotional toll of her advocacy surprised Dorothy. Although most people were kind and appreciative, she could feel a deep anger beneath their fear toward the historic injustice and systemic neglect that left her community vulnerable. Dorothy understood too well.

Centuries of exploitation and firsthand experiences of racism in health care have deepened mistrust of medical research within many Black communities. Historical instances of medical racism, such as the notorious Tuskegee Study[1]—carried out just one hundred miles from Panola by the US Public Health Service—involved physicians and researchers who observed the effects of untreated syphilis on African American men without their informed consent. Even after penicillin was established as the standard treatment in 1943, study investigators withheld this lifesaving medication.[2] This history is the backdrop to ongoing, present-day racial disparities in health care access and treatment that continue to drive hesitancy to engage with health care and medical research.[3] During times of crises like pandemics, these fears can be even more pronounced.

It was a painful and troubling realization: the very people who needed the most support were often the hardest to convince. And help was very much in need; data from trackers such as the COVID Racial Data Tracker[4] showed that Black patients were still dying at four to six times the rate of white patients, regardless of their age, in 2021. Nationwide data from the CDC showed a disheartening pattern that seemed to repeat itself: communities of color that bore the greater burden of COVID hospitalization and death rates were also the ones with lower access to and uptake of the COVID vaccine.[5]

But Dorothy had something that doctors, scientists, political leaders, pharmaceutical companies, and the media didn't have. She had the trust of her community, built over years of shared experiences, genuine connections, a deep understanding of their struggles and fears, and an unshakable commitment to their well-being. These qualities would prove vital to her efforts as she worked to change hearts and minds, mobilize action, and ultimately save lives.

One afternoon, still a few names short of their goal for the mobile vaccine clinic, Dorothy drove to LaDenzel Colvin's house. As she pulled into the driveway, she spotted him in his usual baseball cap and T-shirt. He was getting ready to grill baby back ribs that looked like they had been marinated to perfection with barbeque sauce, tangy vinegar, sweet molasses, and a kick of spice.

"You doin' all right?" she called out. "You had your shot?"

"I just really haven't made my mind up to take it for real," LaDenzel replied doubtfully. He explained that he had gotten COVID already.

"And that wasn't enough for you to make your mind up?" Dorothy laughed, throwing her hands up in mock exasperation. Then, her expression turned serious as she leaned in. "You got to think about this. You see it can hit you, right?"

LaDenzel hesitated, a flicker of concern crossing his face.

Sensing his uncertainty, Dorothy seized the moment. "That's what I'm saying! So . . . can I put you on the list, then?" she asked, her tone warm and encouraging.

"I don't know, Miss Dorothy . . ." He trailed off, glancing back at the grill.

"Ha! I thought I just made your mind up." Dorothy chuckled, her laughter momentarily lightening the mood. She paused, then, her tone turning serious again, she recounted how her nephew's wife had contracted COVID on her birthday, initially thinking it was just a cold.

"She got a little worse every day. On Sunday, she was gone. You can't take no chances," Dorothy said.

LaDenzel's expression shifted. Finally, he let out a sigh. "Yeah, put me down," he called out, somewhat reluctantly as he ran back up his wooden porch steps.

"Good! I'm proud of you." Dorothy smiled, clapping her hands and eyes crinkling with a wide smile that spread across her face.

Later, Dorothy and Drucilla sat on a park bench in the late afternoon sun, surrounded by the comforting sounds of cicadas.

"We have a list of twenty-four people on this sheet, and there are sixteen on this sheet," Drucilla said, looking at their lists.

"So we're right at forty, then," Dorothy said. "Will you try to get everything [to the hospital] tonight or tomorrow?"

"Yes, I'll get them this information tonight."

As the day of the vaccine clinic dawned, cars started to arrive early in the morning. Dorothy stood on the side of the road, pad of paper in hand, diligently checking off names as each person rolled in. She was on a mission to transform every name on her list from a mere pledge into a fully vaccinated individual.

"Hey, Fonda! You ready?" she greeted warmly.

"You still dance like you used to?" Dorothy teased an elderly man. He wore a toffee-brown newsboy cap that perched neatly atop his head, the rich hue complementing the warmth of his weathered complexion, and the white fuzz of his hair poking out just below his cap.

He laughed back. "If they play music, I be dancing."

As the day wore on and droplets of rain started to fall, Dorothy noticed that LaDenzel still hadn't come in. With less than forty minutes left in the clinic, she picked up her cell phone and dialed his number, hoping to hear that he was on his way. No answer.

She shook her head. "Lord have mercy . . . I thought I had him."

With just a few minutes left to spare, LaDenzel drove up in his dark gray Honda.

"Here he comes, y'all! The last one. You made it, then!"

"Yes, ma'am."

"We *glad* you made it. I was scared you got kinda nervous and weren't coming."

"I'm not afraid of a shot," LaDenzel said confidently with a grin.

Dorothy chuckled, smiling behind her mask as the nurse administered the vaccine to his left arm.

"That wasn't so bad now, was it?" Dorothy said. "I bet you barely felt it. Now . . . how did those baby back ribs come out?"

———

By December 2021, Dorothy and Drucilla had successfully convinced all but 5 of the 344 residents in Panola to receive their vaccinations. In stark contrast, Alabama ranked among the states with the lowest vaccination rates in the country, with only 48 percent fully vaccinated and 58 percent having received at least one dose by the end of 2021.[6] Somehow, Dorothy's light shone through, and people beyond Panola noticed, including filmmakers and social justice advocates Rachael DeCruz and Jeremy Levine. After discovering her general store and her passionate efforts to promote vaccine advocacy, they were inspired to create a documentary short film to share her compelling story with the world.[7]

In recognition of her exceptional efforts, she was honored as one of the recipients of the Best of Womankind in 2021, receiving special acknowledgment from Dr. Anthony Fauci at USA TODAY's Best of Humankind

Awards.[8] Fauci praised Dorothy as a "bridge" between her community and essential health resources, highlighting the vital role of trusted local figures in public health initiatives.

Dorothy's relentless dedication also underscores a more profound issue: the systemic gaps and lack of infrastructure, such as inadequate broadband access, unpaved roads, and the absence of a designated local health department, that created an environment where her efforts were not only necessary but truly extraordinary.

While it is both natural and important to celebrate individual heroism, the true takeaway is that we cannot rely on extraordinary individuals to bear the burden of addressing deep-seated structural disadvantages. This approach is neither sustainable nor scalable, and it fails to hold other entities such as government, industry, health care, and academia accountable for their roles in perpetuating systemic disparities. Instead, we can focus on creating comprehensive systems that support and empower communities, ensuring that collective responsibility is shared rather than placed on the shoulders of a few. The downstream solution is to find people like Dorothy; the upstream solution is to improve the places in which Dorothys live.

But improving economic, social, and environmental conditions and strengthening infrastructure takes time and resources. It also requires buy-in from the community and a clear understanding of its unique needs, as every community is different. Blanket policies and one-size-fits-all interventions may not be effective. So where does that leave communities in need right now?

Community-based health interventions can provide support and fill gaps while long-term improvements are underway. These organized efforts aim to enhance the health of communities, actively engaging community members in various ways, from initial involvement to full leadership roles.[9] At their core, community-based approaches invite members to participate in shaping their health trajectory, creating pathways for collaboration and shared decision-making. A meta-analysis of 131 community-engaged health intervention studies showed that engaging community members in public health initiatives significantly improves health behaviors, health outcomes, self-confidence in managing health, and social support among disadvantaged groups.[10] Another meta-review of community-engaged research revealed similar findings, demonstrating significant improvements in community health outcomes and highlighting the critical role of community involvement in tackling health inequities.[11]

What makes this category of public health strategies particularly powerful is their adaptability to the unique context and needs of each community. Strategies can range from collaborative research to grassroots organizing, all beginning with community engagement where local voices are heard and important conversations about health take place in everyday life. It is important to note that the types of community-based strategies discussed in the following sections aren't set in stone; rather, they exist along a continuum where the boundaries can blur.[12] As such, certain activities and elements within these frameworks may overlap, reflecting the complex and dynamic nature of community involvement in health initiatives and the varying needs of different community partnerships.

COMMUNITY ENGAGEMENT

Community engagement and valuing community input are cornerstones of building trust and collaboration, often serving as the first step for those seeking to partner with and learn from local populations. This process involves engaging community members in discussions and activities that affect their health, focusing on the importance of building ongoing relationships and having open dialogue. Community engagement, however, does not necessarily involve community members in the decision-making or design of research initiatives, and there may not be a specific health intervention involved at all. At this basic level of community involvement, the focus is on fostering connections, gathering valuable input, and raising awareness about health issues. In this process, community members are not passive recipients of information or resources; they are encouraged to share their perspectives and experiences, which can help shape future health initiatives. Research shows that when communities feel genuinely engaged, they are more likely to participate in health programs, advocate for their own needs, and experience improved health and reduced health inequities.[13]

The Latinos en Control intervention, developed by researchers at the University of Massachusetts Medical School, exemplifies how community input can be instrumental to the success of health programs. Designed to enhance diabetes management among low-income Latinos with type

2 diabetes, this culturally tailored initiative began with researchers engaging with the community to understand their perspectives and identify specific needs and preferences.[14] Drawing from this valuable feedback, the researchers developed an intensive yearlong program using elements such as visual aids to simplify complex concepts, engaging activities like "foods bingo" and cooking lessons, and the use of popular media, such as educational soap operas, to help participants better manage their diabetes.[15] The intervention was rigorously tested through a randomized trial, resulting in improvements in several health indicators, including reductions in average blood glucose levels, improved diet, increased blood glucose self-monitoring, and decreased depressive symptoms.[16]

Another exemplary health initiative that benefited from community engagement is the Community Healthy Activities Model Program for Seniors. Developed by researchers at the University of California San Francisco, this program started as a demonstration project focused on promoting physical activity among seniors living in low-income housing. Researchers engaged seniors to gather their perspectives on activities designed to boost physical activity and to learn their preferences for program formats. This collaboration informed the design of an intervention that successfully increased physical activity among older adults.[17] Over time, the program evolved through rigorous scientific studies and scalable adaptations, integrating feedback from community agencies across San Francisco. These local organizations were crucial in tailoring the physical activity intervention to meet the unique needs and preferences of their neighborhoods. For instance, initiatives such as "Seniors in Motion for Health" and "Siempre Activo" were specifically adapted by organizations committed to serving their respective communities. This resulted in increased physical activity across multiple communities, with several peer-reviewed studies documenting the program's success.[18]

COMMUNITY CENTERING

Community centering takes engagement a step further by systematically incorporating community input into the design and delivery of predefined health programs or initiatives. Though researchers lead these types of initiatives, community members have a stronger, active role in shaping community-centered interventions and may take the lead on certain elements. The focus is on collaboratively developing interventions designed to address the needs, cultural values, and available resources of the community. By actively engaging community members in the planning process, these interventions become more relevant to their needs, leading to higher acceptance, increased likelihood of community participation, and greater health benefits.

One nationwide initiative that integrates community-centric strategies is the Community Engagement Alliance Against COVID-19 (CEAL). The National Institutes of Health (NIH) initially created the initiative to increase recruitment of marginalized racial and ethnic groups in clinical trials and vaccine efforts to reduce racial disparities in COVID.[19] CEAL cultivated community partnerships through community listening sessions, workshops, seminars, and other community forums to gather feedback and refining strategies from community partners.[20] Community-centered strategies included conducting a listening tour in Mississippi with Black community members,[21] producing an animated video with local artists in Louisiana to encourage trial participation among communities of color,[22] and working with Arizona's community health workers and promoters to increase awareness and trust in COVID-19 messaging.[23] This federal initiative has since expanded its focus to address broader health disparities, including maternal health and climate health, through community-centric partnerships.

Another example of a community-centered approach is the Brookings Supports Breastfeeding initiative, which aims to increase breastfeeding rates among mothers.[24] This collaborative effort involved a partnership between South Dakota State University researchers, the Brookings Area Chamber of Commerce, the Brookings Health System, and local breastfeeding advocates and families. The initiative used public deliberation to gather feedback from local families, ensuring that the program components aligned with their needs and preferences. The resulting initiative included partnering with local businesses to support breastfeeding employees and customers; improving hospital breastfeeding resources through a Brookings Health System's Baby-Friendly designation; and establishing the New Beginnings Baby Café, a free support group led by lactation consultants. Research showed that this community-centric, multisectoral approach was vital for increasing broader awareness and community-level support for breastfeeding in work, community, and health care settings, reinforcing the idea that centering community needs and values can pave the way for improved health behaviors and outcomes.[25]

COMMUNITY EMPOWERMENT

Community empowerment emphasizes deeper community involvement and capacity building, enabling communities to lead their own initiatives. Community empowerment is a process that enhances the capacity of individuals and groups within a community to make informed decisions, advocate for their needs, and take action to improve their health and well-being.[26] It involves equipping community members with the knowledge, skills, and resources necessary to influence the conditions that affect their lives.[27] Community members collaborate with researchers and organizations to take on leadership roles in identifying health issues, developing and implementing solutions, and engaging in advocacy efforts for health initiatives.

One compelling example of community health empowerment is the Communities in Control Study, which examined residents' health outcomes across 150 disadvantaged areas of England through the Big Local program.[28] This initiative allocated over £1 million to each neighborhood, empowering communities to set their own priorities, determine how to use the funding to improve their communities, and address historical funding disparities. Residents improved their communities in various ways, such as funding community gardens, organizing social events to foster connections, improving public spaces, supporting local businesses, addressing specific health needs, enhancing education programs, and creating safe play areas for children, reflecting their unique priorities and aspirations for community development. Research revealed significant improvements in mental well-being, particularly among those who felt a sense of collective control, highlighting the impact of resident engagement in decision-making.[29] Overall, residents experienced positive outcomes, and although results varied by location, the program's benefits on average outweighed its costs.

Another notable initiative is the community empowerment-based response to HIV among sex workers, led by researchers from Johns Hopkins

Bloomberg School of Public Health.[30] This program recognizes that addressing HIV in these vulnerable populations requires understanding and tackling the broader contexts that heighten their risk of infection. Empowerment strategies that targeted capacity building and skill building included training sex workers on HIV prevention and health advocacy, establishing peer-led support networks, engaging sex workers in advocacy and outreach efforts to address systemic health issues, and providing access to essential resources like condoms and health care services. A systematic review of empowerment approaches has shown protective effects against HIV and STI infections,[31] demonstrating how equipping people with knowledge, resources, and skills can meaningfully improve health.

Storytelling is another powerful tool that can empower communities by linking health messages to everyday experiences, allowing adults and children alike to share personal narratives that connect to broader health issues.[32] This approach especially resonates with underresourced and marginalized populations by helping them acknowledge structural barriers to health while highlighting their own resources and strengths. Through these shared stories, storytellers are inspired to make positive changes in their lives and communities.

My team's research on the H2GO! program focused on empowering low-income youth to drink less sugary drinks, stay hydrated with water, and promote healthy weight gain through youth-produced narratives.[33] Developed collaboratively with Boys and Girls Club (BGC) staff, parents, and children in Massachusetts, the intervention featured interactive, group-based learning sessions led by BGC staff, incorporating activities such as blinded taste tests, sugar measurement demonstrations, beverage scavenger hunts at local stores, and critically analyzing sugary drink advertisements. In addition, the program's youth-led activities guided participants to create their own messages and narratives on swapping out sugary drinks for water through various media (print, audio, or video) which they then shared with their families, fostering a deeper connection to the program and enhancing their role as health advocates within their homes. The intervention concluded with a youth-led Club night, where participants displayed their narratives and organized a flavored water taste test for their peers, complete with prizes like reusable water bottles, fruit infuser water bottles, and sparkling water machines. This engaging youth-led community event created a fun atmosphere that encouraged healthy choices and empowered youth to take ownership of their health advocacy efforts.

Our randomized study showed that children and parents who participated in the program had significant health improvements over six months. Children became confident in their ability to make healthy choices, drank less sugary drinks, drank more water, and experienced healthier weight growth compared to a control group.[34] Although parents were indirect beneficiaries of the H2GO! program, they also reported improvements in their own health habits over six months, including reduced consumption of sugary drinks and increased water intake. The success of empowerment interventions like H2GO! highlights the transformative potential of community members, including youth, as leaders in health initiatives, cultivating a supportive environment for collective action and promoting healthier lifestyles from within.

COMMUNITY-BASED PARTICIPATORY RESEARCH

Community-Based Participatory Research (CBPR) is a research paradigm that involves community members as equal partners in the research process to target health disparities.[35] In CBPR, community members and researchers engage in shared decision-making and mutual respect to address the community's needs and priorities at every stage of research, leading to more relevant and effective health solutions.[36] This partnership allows both parties to codevelop research questions and strategies that reflect the community's concerns and aspirations and lead to impactful, sustainable solutions rooted in community and cultural strengths. A systematic review of CBPR interventions targeting diabetes found that 14 out of 16 studies showed significant improvements in key health metrics, such as average blood sugar (glucose) levels and blood pressure.[37]

A specific example of CBPR is the Strong Heart Study, which focuses on cardiovascular disease among American Indian men and women. Launched in 1984, this ongoing cohort study is the largest epidemiologic investigation of heart disease in American Indians, involving participants from thirteen tribal nations across Arizona, Oklahoma, North Dakota, and South Dakota.[38] Throughout the study, researchers have followed the

CBPR model, ensuring that community members are involved in all stages of research design and implementation. Through CBPR, the Strong Heart Study identified health barriers such as limited budgets and lack of access to fresh produce. In response, researchers collaborated with community members to develop and test health interventions addressing these needs, while also providing pilot grants for research initiatives led by community members to support tribal health programs.[39] These collaborations have generated hundreds of peer-reviewed publications that offer valuable insights into improving the health of American Indian populations.[40] Notably, partnerships formed during the study have strengthened relationships between researchers and tribal communities, fostering long-term trust and collaboration that extend beyond the study itself.

Another example of applying CBPR is Weaving an Islander Network for Cancer Awareness, Research, and Training (WINCART), which addressed cancer health disparities among Pacific Islanders in California. Funded by the National Cancer Institute, this project involved collaboration between researchers from five universities and eight community-based organizations serving Chamorro, Marshallese, Native Hawaiians, Samoans, and Tongans.[41] WINCART embraced cooperative engagement to foster co-learning, capacity building, and the promotion of culturally relevant cancer awareness and prevention strategies within Pacific Islander communities. Research findings show that WINCART demonstrated progress in increasing cancer awareness and screening, reducing tobacco health disparities, and increasing physical activity levels among Pacific Islander communities.[42]

COMMUNITY-DRIVEN INTERVENTIONS

At the highest level of community involvement are *community-driven interventions*, where local residents take the lead in addressing their health challenges, while researchers and other organizations may play a supporting, funding, or technical-assistance role. This approach emphasizes local ownership and leadership, empowering communities to create their own solutions. Community members are the primary decision-makers who identify pressing health issues, set priorities, and design programs that reflect their aspirations. This approach motivates individuals to invest in the success of the initiatives they help create. Dorothy's COVID-19 vaccine effort is Panola's shining example.

Other examples include Kaiser Permanente's HEAL Zones, a community-driven initiative aimed at promoting healthy eating and active living in communities across Southern California.[43] By partnering with public health departments, community organizations, schools, and advocacy groups, HEAL Zones empower local residents to tackle disparities in chronic diseases like diabetes and heart disease. Local leaders take the lead in designing and implementing programs that encourage healthier diets and physical activity, while Kaiser Permanente supports these efforts by providing technical assistance and expertise. This partnership cultivates a collaborative environment that leverages the complementary strengths of different stakeholders to create impactful health solutions.

To promote health, each HEAL Zone focuses on small, low-income communities of ten thousand to twenty thousand residents, all grappling with high rates of obesity and chronic diseases. Within these zones, community coalitions are empowered to organize, create, and implement tailored strategies that address local needs, instilling a sense of ownership among residents over health initiatives. This community-driven initiative has rolled out over 230 strategies designed to improve policies and programs for healthy eating and physical activity and transform the environment to make healthier choices the default option. Research indicates that HEAL communities with sustained investment in these strategies have experienced significant improvements in health behaviors.[44] Such examples demonstrate the profound impact of grassroots, community-driven interventions. When people are positioned to lead and supported with resources, they can create meaningful change within their communities.

The success of community-based initiatives requires funding and support from a wide array of stakeholders. These include local health advocacy groups that provide grassroots support; foundations that can fund innovative projects; academic or research institutions that can contribute evaluation or analytic skills; health care systems that can implement community health programs and offer medical resources; government entities that can provide policy support and funding through local, state, and federal agencies; and business and industry partners who can contribute resources and sponsorship for community initiatives.

Local funding can make a big difference to communities by empowering grassroots solutions. For example, the Robert Wood Johnson Foundation's annual "Culture of Health Prize" recognizes innovative, community-led health initiatives.[45] In 2023, winners included Go Austin/Vamos Austin, which secured childcare resources to support working families and successfully advocated to make flood insurance more affordable for low-income families, and the Detroit Association of Black Organizations, which united over 130 organizations to provide health screenings, after-school programs, and suicide prevention efforts.[46] In northern Minnesota, the Fond du Lac Band of Lake Superior Chippewa revitalized traditional farming to enhance food sovereignty, supporting school meals and combating diabetes while reconnecting Band members with their cultural heritage.[47]

Investing in community-driven initiatives such as these harnesses the unique needs and strengths of each population, cultivating a culture of health deeply rooted in local contexts. Support from a variety of stakeholders, including foundations, government entities, local organizations, and community members, plays a crucial role in catalyzing and sustaining these initiatives through financial resources, technical assistance, social capital, or policy backing.

Whether through engagement, centering, empowerment, participatory action, or community-driven approaches, the spectrum from initial involvement to ownership demonstrates the transformative potential of community interventions. By recognizing and valuing the voices of community members, we can create more effective and sustainable health solutions that address specific needs. These collaborative efforts illuminate a path toward lasting change, showcasing the power of connection, cooperation, and collective action. Dorothy's love for her community exemplifies this spirit.

"They look to me," she said. "Every community needs a leader who cares. Don't think you can't make a difference. Do what you can to help your community; it will help you find the light in the dark."

CHAPTER 10

The Collective Cure

Back in the summer of 2013, the pilot hybrid course for the physician students at Harvard was well underway. Each week from June to July, I released an online module on a different social or structural determinant of health for them to complete, synthesizing many of the materials and concepts you've just encountered in this book. Students applied these ideas to their own work in a course blog, where I provided individual and collective feedback.

As the weeks passed, I noticed a shift in the atmosphere. The initial skepticism began to melt away. Even the student who had publicly warned me that first day, doubt written all over his face, was among the first to send an email of encouragement. One by one, they expressed how much they enjoyed the online modules and—most importantly—the content we were covering.

By the time I met them again in person for on-site seminars on August 1, the room felt transformed—warmer, lighter—as if curiosity and genuine engagement had replaced the palpable reservation just three months earlier. By the end of the course, the change in mood was unmistakable. Course evaluations came in: a 4.8 out of 5 for overall course quality and effectiveness in teaching.

"Monica really surprised us and exceeded our expectations!"

"The material is very relevant if not essential for today's health care executives."

It seemed both the course and I had surprised them. What I didn't expect was how the students would surprise me. Some students shared how they had already begun applying the material through integrating social determinants into clinic protocols, revisiting their hospital's community outreach strategies to improve cancer screenings, or designing policies targeting mental health among health care professionals. Others sought guidance after the course concluded on designing and evaluating population health strategies.

One student, now a prominent president of a major health care system, wrote: "Your course on social determinants of population health had a profound impact on me. There's simply no other way to say it. I hope to use what I've learned to implement programs that emphasize prevention and proactive approaches."

Of course, there were still a few who didn't see the relevance of the course to their work. But for every skeptic, there were many more who embraced the material and carried it forward. I've come to realize that my goal isn't to change every mind. Sometimes, all it takes is one person seeing the world a bit differently to spark a ripple effect that reaches far beyond what we originally imagined.

What started as a pilot hybrid course in 2013 soon became a core course of the MHCM program. Over the years, it has grown, reaching nearly 400 health care leaders from the US and abroad across 14 cohorts and counting, spanning four US presidential administrations, and continuing through the challenges of a global pandemic and heightened social and political division. I still teach the course today, refining it each year to evolve alongside the world it seeks to impact as new evidence, challenges, and opportunities emerge. And with it, the mission and journey remain the same: to bring the vital lens of social determinants to curious minds everywhere.

Teaching this course also helped me more fully appreciate an important truth: health care professionals cannot tackle the root causes of poor health alone. They do not have the resources, capacity, or authority—nor should we expect them to. They are trained to care for patients, not to dismantle the systemic inequities that occur outside hospital walls. While they can meet patients where they are with a deeper understanding of their social, economic, and environmental circumstances, real change requires more than a partnership between public health and medicine (believe me, I'm married to a doctor).

Public health, by its nature, is a shared responsibility. It extends far beyond the realm of health care to include housing, education, employment, urban planning, and more. Creating better health for all requires collective action across these sectors, an ecosystem working in concert to create conditions where every community can thrive. It's not just about treating illness; it's about building systems that make better health possible for all. This vision calls on each of us to recognize our role in this larger public health ecosystem, where personal *and* collective responsibility is reflected in policy and initiatives, as well as embodied in the way some communities already support one another.

During my time supporting La Danza Huitzilmeztli, I saw how a community can come together as a seamless, interconnected system, where every individual plays a vital role in contributing to community well-being. Under the open skies, La Danza unfolded as a beautiful, multigenerational collaboration with women at its center. Elders, mothers, and young women played central roles as dancers, supported by firekeepers, childcare providers, and meal preparers who ensured that the women could fully engage in their sacred work.

While the dancers moved gracefully in their rituals late into the night, firekeepers tended the sacred flames, ensuring they burned strong and steady over four days and four nights. Childcare providers cared for the little ones day and night, creating a space for mothers to focus on their roles as dancers. In the kitchen, Abuela Xochi oversaw the preparation of nourishing meals made from scratch, using fresh produce from local farms. Meanwhile, supporters in the kitchen, including me, chopped, diced, cleaned, organized, and kept everything running smoothly to feed the community.

In the medicine tent, trained providers offered teas, ointments, and traditional remedies to restore balance and energy to those in need of care. Supporters woke around midnight to accompany dancers as they moved until sunrise, swaying and praying alongside them and sharing in the ceremonial pipe. Every role was essential, valued, and carefully structured. These interdependent efforts created a community where everyone contributed, reinforcing the collective harmony that sustained La Danza.

This deeply collaborative approach mirrors the efforts required for strong public health. Just as the La Danza community recognized the importance of individual contributions to sustain their shared rituals, addressing the root causes of health and disease necessitates a similarly integrated ecosystem. La Danza also reminded me that collective responsibility goes beyond simply completing tasks; it's also about valuing the relationships and interdependence that support us. On a broader scale, the Green & Healthy Homes Initiative exemplifies how sectors such as housing, education, employment, urban planning, and health care each play a vital role in creating healthier communities. Public health thrives when every sector acknowledges and respects each other's role, inviting collaboration to create environments where everyone has a fair opportunity to lead a healthy life.

This approach embodies the upstream vision of addressing social determinants of health, creating the conditions for people to thrive physically, emotionally, socially, and spiritually. Public health often focuses on the "what" of health, the treatments and metrics. But La Danza reminds us to focus on the "how" and "why" of care. How and why we care for people matters as much as what we provide. When health care is integrated with holistic, culturally sensitive, and community-driven approaches, it becomes more than a service—it becomes a lifeline that addresses the full spectrum of human need.

When we look upstream, we see that true change isn't about isolated efforts or simply scaling interventions proven in controlled environments. It's about creating an integrated system, much like La Danza itself, where collective responsibility and holistic care are embedded in daily life. This vision calls on leaders across public health, government, education, business, and urban planning to collaborate and commit to building environments where healthy, thriving communities can take root.

An ambitious vision, yes, but one that is not without precedent. Consider "Blue Zones," regions of the world where people consistently live significantly longer and healthier lives.[1] The term was popularized by Dan Buettner and his team, whose research identified five regions with remarkably high concentrations of centenarians: Okinawa, Japan; Ikaria, Greece; Sardinia, Italy; Nicoya, Costa Rica; and Loma Linda, California.[2] In these regions, it is common for individuals to live active and fulfilling lives well into their nineties and even beyond one hundred years. While genetics undoubtedly play a role, research has shown that the Blue Zones phenomenon is primarily driven by lifestyle, community structure, environmental factors, and social connections[3]—many of the very social and structural determinants we have explored in this book.

Studies of Blue Zones reveal key factors that promote longevity and health, such as regular physical activity embedded in daily routines, plant-based diets with minimal processed foods, strong social networks, and a sense of purpose or "ikigai," as the Japanese call it.[4] For example, research shows that communities in Okinawa, Japan, benefit from *moais* (small, close-knit social groups that provide mutual support throughout life).[5] In Sardinia, Italy, the shepherding lifestyle embeds walking across hilly terrain into everyday life, which promotes cardiovascular health and muscular endurance well into old age.[6]

In Icaria, Greece, walking isn't exercise—it's a way of life. Pedestrian-friendly pathways connect neighborhoods, shops, and gathering spaces, seamlessly weaving movement into daily routines. Whether strolling to the market or visiting a neighbor, residents naturally boost their cardiovascular health while strengthening social bonds.[7] The concept of Blue Zones illustrates a critical point: when communities are intentionally structured to support healthy behaviors, better health outcomes follow naturally.

But what maintains health in already healthy places isn't the same as what's needed to shift the health of an entire community or population facing significant challenges. Recognizing this, Dan Buettner and his team developed Blue Zones Project sites to apply the lessons of longevity to other communities.[8] Project sites have unmet health needs and undergo a structured intervention, with the goal of replicating established health-promoting elements in a new location. Communities are carefully chosen through a detailed selection process that assesses their readiness to embrace change, level of local engagement, and existing health data.

To become a certified Blue Zones Community, a community must have broad and committed buy-in. To qualify, communities must meet specific benchmarks across sectors: at least 20 percent of residents must sign a Blue Zones Personal Pledge, committing to small but impactful lifestyle changes; 50 percent of the top 20 employers must adopt Blue Zones Worksite practices to promote workplace wellness; 25 percent of independently owned restaurants must embrace healthier dining as Blue Zones Restaurants; 25 percent of public schools and grocery stores must integrate Blue Zones principles; and the community must complete a comprehensive Community Policy Pledge to align local policies with health-focused goals. Additionally, a sustainable funding source must be secured to position these efforts for long-term success.[9] To date, there are a dozen Blue Zone Project communities in North America.[10]

Though each community faces unique health needs, resources, and challenges, every Blue Zones Project is built on common core pillars: policy change, environmental design, and community support and connection. This multifaceted, community-centered approach weaves together reformative policies, thoughtfully designed spaces, and community practices. By addressing health from these interconnected angles, Blue Zones Projects cultivate wellness that extends beyond individuals to uplift entire communities.[11]

ENVIRONMENTAL DESIGN AND PUBLIC SPACES

A cornerstone of Blue Zones Project sites is environmental redesign, which encourages physical activity and social engagement through intentionally designed public spaces. In Sardinia, narrow, walkable streets encourage residents to remain active throughout their lives, while the strong tradition of social gatherings in central plazas reinforces community bonds. Similarly, in Ikaria and Okinawa, abundant public spaces facilitate outdoor activities such as walking, gardening, and celebrating festivals, creating opportunities for both physical health and emotional connection.

Blue Zones Project sites in the US have adopted these principles to transform environments where health-promoting spaces are scarce. Albert Lea, Minnesota, the first certified Blue Zones Project site in the US,[12] serves as a standout example of a community that embraced walkability to improve health. Throughout its transformation, the city added over 10 miles of sidewalks and bike lanes and increased trail usage by 38 percent. Streets were made safer with crosswalks, better lighting, and traffic-calming measures, creating a pedestrian-friendly environment that encouraged outdoor activity and social interaction.

The improvements in health were stunning: between 2010 and 2016, the community saw a 35 percent drop in smoking, a 12 percent decline in high cholesterol, a 4 percent decrease in high blood pressure, and a 2.9

years projected increase in lifespan.[13] Residents also reported a 14 percent increase in fresh produce consumption and a 12 percent rise in community pride. Community-level changes in Albert Lea also had a measurable economic benefit, including $8.6 million in projected health care cost savings for local employers, a 34 percent drop in health insurance claims for a regional energy company, and double-digit growth in fresh produce and water sales at local grocery stores.

Beyond Blue Zones, work around the world shows how redesigning and "re-naturing" environments can improve health. For instance, Seoul, South Korea, restored the Cheonggyecheon Stream by dismantling an elevated highway and restoring the historical stream below.[14] This restoration project transformed a previously congested and polluted area into an ecologically sensitive green corridor, featuring ample pedestrian pathways and twenty-two new bridges. The stream restoration yielded significant environmental, health, and economic benefits, including improved air quality and resulting respiratory health, enhanced biodiversity, reduced urban heat effects, increased public transportation use, and stimulation of business growth and property values.

In Melbourne, Australia, the Urban Forest Strategy aims to increase tree canopy coverage from 22 percent to 40 percent by 2040 to combat urban heatwaves.[15] Studies show that increasing tree coverage in urban areas offers numerous health benefits, including reduced heat stress, improved air quality, lower rates of cardiovascular disease, decreased stress levels, and increased physical activity due to more walkable environments.[16] Philadelphia has also set a goal of reaching 30 percent canopy coverage in each neighborhood by 2025. A health-impact assessment estimated that reaching this goal could prevent about 403 premature deaths in the city annually, with 244 of these in lower socioeconomic areas.[17] Such efforts show how planting trees and creating green spaces can produce numerous economic, environmental, health, and societal benefits.

In 2010, Mexico City introduced the Ecobici bike-share program, which gives residents access to bicycles for short trips across the city.[18] Having started with 85 stations and 1,114 bicycles, the Ecobici has grown into Latin America's largest bicycle-sharing program, boasting 687 stations and 9,308 bicycles as of July 2022.[19] Funded by the Mexico City government and managed by the Secretariat of the Environment, Ecobici has become an integral part of the city's transportation network, promoting sustainable mobility, reducing traffic congestion, and decreasing air pollution. Participants report improved physical activity, cardiovascular fitness, and respiratory health.[20] These examples illustrate the power of improving our environments and the way we navigate them to enhance health on a large scale.

POLICY CHANGES FOR HEALTHIER LIVING

Another cornerstone of Blue Zones Projects is policy reform—creating rules and frameworks that make healthier choices the norm. These policies prioritize walkability, access to nutritious foods, and opportunities for social connection, shaping environments where well-being is built into daily life.

In 2014, Fort Worth, Texas, ranked among the nation's lowest metro areas for well-being. Texas Health and city leaders launched permanent policy and social network changes across worksites, schools, and community spaces to make healthier choices easier.[21] The city introduced policies that incentivized grocery stores to open in underserved neighborhoods, significantly expanding access to fresh fruits and vegetables for thousands of residents in food deserts. Other policy changes further cemented the project's impact, such as smoke-free city parks and workplaces, combined with $6.2 million invested in Safe Routes to School infrastructure and the introduction of electric buses.[22] More than 88,000 residents engaged in project programs, contributing to a 14 percent rise in those who describe themselves as "thriving" and an 8.8 percent increase in civic pride.

The health impact was substantial: from 2014 to 2018, the city achieved a 31 percent reduction in smoking, an 11 percent drop in high cholesterol, and a 7 percent decrease in high blood pressure, while exercise rates rose by 17 percent and fresh produce consumption increased by 3 percent. Overall well-being scores climbed by 3.7 points, elevating Fort Worth's metro area ranking a whopping 127 spots (from 185th to 58th) out of nearly 190 regions. Employers also reported financial benefits. For example, the Dallas Fort Worth International Airport saw its health care cost increases grow at a rate 40 percent lower than the national average, and Mother Parkers Tea & Coffee reported a 16 percent drop in medical claims and a 26 percent reduction in pharmacy claims in just one year.[23] To date, Fort Worth is the country's largest Blue Zones–certified community, exemplifying how public-private partnerships can reshape health and well-being on a citywide scale.

Health-promoting policies elsewhere have also demonstrated the power of legislative change. A meta-analysis of 62 studies evaluating the global impact of sugary drink taxes found that such measures led to an average 15 percent reduction in sugary drink sales.[24] In 2017, Philadelphia implemented a beverage tax on sugar-sweetened drinks,[25] following the precedent set by Berkeley, California.[26] Evaluations of these specific city-level taxes have found reductions in sugary drink consumption by as much as 35–50 percent.[27] The taxes also raised significant funds that were reinvested into community initiatives. For example, Philadelphia's 1.5-cents-per-ounce tax on sugary beverages has generated about $409 million from 2017 to 2024.[28] Nearly 40 percent of this revenue—about $158 million—has been allocated to fund the city's free prekindergarten program, expanding access to early childhood education. The remaining funds have supported community schools and the revitalization of parks, recreation centers, and libraries.

In the realm of road safety, mandatory seat belt laws and accompanying public education campaigns enacted across the US starting in the 1980s significantly improved traffic safety. By 2020, seat belt use exceeded 90 percent nationwide, a substantial increase from 14 percent in 1983,[29] preventing about 15,000 deaths and 375,000 serious injuries each year.[30]

Overseas, Finland's salt reduction legislative and campaign efforts provide a striking example of how focused policies can improve population health. In the 1970s, Finland initiated a community-based salt reduction campaign to combat high cardiovascular disease rates that united health organizations, schools, media, and the food industry.[31] Following its success, the program expanded nationwide. In 1993, Finland implemented mandatory salt-labeling legislation, requiring high-sodium foods to display their salt content by weight and include a "high salt content" warning.[32] This policy, combined with public awareness campaigns and media support, significantly shifted societal attitudes toward salt consumption. Over two decades, these efforts led to a 40 percent reduction in average salt intake and a 75–80 percent decrease in deaths from stroke and heart disease.[33]

In Bogotá, Colombia, the innovative public policy Ciclovía initiative began transforming urban life as early as 1974.[34] Each Sunday, the city closes over 100 kilometers (62.1 miles) of city streets to motorized traffic, creating safe spaces for pedestrians, cyclists, and skaters. More than two million residents participate weekly, promoting physical activity, reducing air pollution, and fostering a stronger sense of community. Over fifty years later, Ciclovía continues and has since inspired more than 400 cities around the world to follow suit.[35] The enduring success of Ciclovía demonstrates that transitioning away from car dependence is feasible, public spaces can be used to cultivate healthier cities and citizens, and streets can be designed to connect people and build a cohesive urban community.

These examples show that policy changes are more than abstract ideas—they are powerful tools for improving the health of entire populations. Thoughtful policies paired with awareness campaigns can remove barriers to health and foster communities where healthy living becomes the norm. As Blue Zones Project sites and other policy initiatives illustrate, these structural shifts pave the way for long-term improvements in health, proving that *how* we live has as much influence on our health as *where* we live.

BUILDING SOCIAL AND COMMUNITY CONNECTIONS

Another essential pillar of Blue Zones is community connection, emphasizing the importance of social relationships, support, and capital in fostering long-term health and well-being. In Nicoya, Costa Rica, close-knit, multigenerational households naturally support one another, sharing resources, caregiving responsibilities, and healthy habits.[36] In Okinawa, the tradition of forming moais has been linked to higher levels of happiness, lower rates of depression, and extended life expectancy.[37] These deep-rooted cultural practices reflect how tightly woven social bonds improve both individual and community health.

Blue Zones–inspired projects in the US have adapted these principles by cultivating community engagement to achieve collective health goals. In Fort Worth, Texas, numerous faith-based communities participated in the Blue Zones Project by organizing "walking moais," inspired by Okinawan traditions, bringing together small groups of residents for regular walks, providing physical activity and opportunities to build friendships. Communities also organized healthy potlucks, plant-based cooking demonstrations, purpose workshops, and yoga and movement programs. These activities strengthened social bonds, improved mental and physical health, and reduced stress.[38]

In Beach Cities, California (a cluster of cities including Redondo Beach, Hermosa Beach, and Manhattan Beach), the Blue Zones Project also sparked the formation of walking moais for fitness, friendship, and fun. Additionally, Beach Cities created volunteer networks to encourage residents to give back to their community, further deepening ties and reinforcing a culture of collective care. This combined with other environmental and policy initiatives contributed to a 68 percent reduction in childhood obesity, 25 percent drop in adult overweight, 36 percent drop in smoking, 4 percent decrease in daily stress levels, 8 percent increase in exercise, and 6 percent increase in fresh produce consumption from 2010 to 2017.[39]

The power of community engagement and connection extends to other regions as well. In Chicago, Illinois, the "Good Neighbor Campaign" by the Chicago Department of Public Health encouraged residents to check in on elderly neighbors, form support groups, and assist with tasks like prescription pickup.[40] During the COVID-19 pandemic, this campaign played a critical role in reducing isolation, increasing vaccination rates, and fostering a network of care.

In Australia, the Men's Shed movement provides another compelling example of how fostering social connections can improve health.[41] Men's Sheds are community spaces where men gather to work on hands-on projects like woodworking, gardening, or repairing equipment, while also engaging in conversations and mutual support. The initiative largely targets older men, who often experience isolation after retirement or the loss of a spouse. Men's Sheds have expanded globally, demonstrating the universal appeal and efficacy of addressing isolation through communal, purpose-driven spaces. Research indicates that Men's Sheds can have a significant impact, with participants reporting improved mental well-being, reduced loneliness, increased sense of purpose and belonging, and decreased depressive symptoms and thoughts of suicide.[42] Another study reported physical health benefits, including increased mobility, decreased sedentary behavior, improved resilience to physical illness or injury, improved diet, and reduced alcohol consumption.[43] These examples demonstrate that engaging and building community, whether within Blue Zones or beyond, are possible and fundamental to building healthier, more resilient populations.

While each of the strategies of policy, environment, and community can be effective on their own, the greatest impact comes from integration. Communities that embrace all three didn't just improve health and reduce health care costs—they redefined what it means to live well. These case studies demonstrate that healthy, thriving communities are achievable when we adopt a holistic, upstream approach to public health. As a growing body of research shows, the path to better health starts with reimagining how we live, work, and connect—together.

So, how do we get everyone on board to make this vision a reality? A critical part of the answer lies in how we communicate about public health, especially to those who may not immediately understand or embrace the research behind social determinants of health. Sharing data and scientific findings alone isn't enough; it's the stories we tell that truly connect people on a human level to these broader concepts. The language we use and the narratives we craft in sharing research have the power to shift attitudes, change minds, and drive decisions.

This is something I was reminded of when I met Melvin Carter, the forty-sixth mayor of St. Paul, Minnesota, during the 2019 Harvard Business School's Young American Leaders Program. Melvin spoke passionately about transforming his city, not by pushing traditional political levers but by investing in libraries, creating public spaces, and funding job training programs.

A fourth-generation resident, Mayor Carter implemented transformative initiatives: raising the city's minimum wage to $15 per hour, eliminating library late fines, tripling recreational programming, and expanding support for immigrants.[44] His CollegeBound Saint Paul program ensures that every child born in the city starts life with a $50 college savings account. In addition, Mayor Carter launched a $3 million public safety initiative focused on youth employment, mental health, housing support, and violence prevention. His approach blends restorative justice and social workers alongside police officers, aiming to support those in crisis with compassion and care. He wasn't focused on quick fixes; he was planting seeds for long-term, meaningful change.

After his talk, I approached him, excited and energized. "It's so refreshing to hear a politician talk about the social determinants of health!" I said.

He looked back at me with genuine surprise and a touch of bemusement. "Now where did you hear me talk about the social determinants of health?" he asked.

In that moment, I realized that leaders like Mayor Carter understood, perhaps intuitively, that investing in communities through policy, environment, and community shapes health at its roots—even if they don't use the term "social determinants."

Maybe those of us in public health and academia have been approaching it from too narrow a perspective. We often frame health as the ultimate goal. Yes, health is a vital part of the larger puzzle that makes up a full and meaningful life, but it's not the only picture that emerges when the pieces come together. Safe affordable housing, quality education, a livable income, stable employment, clean air and water, access to affordable fresh food, and a sense of belonging in a trusted community—these are cornerstone pieces, fitting together to create a complete picture of well-being. When each piece is in place, we don't just exist; we live, building a life with purpose and connection that is possible *because* health is the foundational backdrop.

Whatever is front and center in the picture is up to each individual. It can be the families and friendships we build, the careers we embark on, the places we explore, the causes we champion, and the hobbies that give us joy. Each of these pursuits becomes possible, reaching its fullest potential, when our health is strong and supported by the broader conditions in which we live.

Perhaps the mayor's response was the most upstream message of all: it's not simply about health—it's about creating the conditions for all of us to thrive. A vision that is both undeniably bold and possible. And the ripple effects of even small changes start with one person, one action, one commitment to move upstream.

Let's get to work.

The Stories We Share

This book began as an idea tossed around during a conversation in 2021, a time when the cracks in our health systems were laid bare for all to see. I had recently joined the Boston University Center for Antiracist Research as the associate director of narrative, working alongside Dr. Ibram X. Kendi. In one of our meetings, I proposed writing a series of op-eds to explain the history and research behind the health inequities that COVID-19 had amplified so starkly.

"How about a book?" Ibram suggested.

I laughed, thinking he was joking. "Who's going to write it?"

"Not me," he said with a smile. Then, with a light but purposeful tone, he added, "You might want to think about connecting your personal story to the research, especially regarding anti-Asian racism. Has it been personal for you?"

The question landed like a stone in my chest. My answer tumbled out before I could think: "It's incredibly personal. I was born in Wuhan."

As I said it, I realized I hadn't talked about my birthplace with anyone new since 2020. At that moment, Ibram's suggestion became something much larger: an invitation to document real stories and truly share them. It was then, in 2021, that I knew this project would be about much more than summarizing research. It would be about stories—stories that could make the invisible visible, the systemic personal, and the academic accessible. It would also be about re-opening chapters of my own life that I hadn't fully explored, and confronting the ways the COVID-19 pandemic intersected with my identity as a Chinese American woman and my profession as a public health expert, born in the very city that had been spotlighted on the global stage.

The journey of writing this book meant revisiting painful memories and unearthing the collective trauma borne by so many throughout our lifespans. But it also became a way to celebrate the strength of those who believe in a better world and refuse to let their voices be silenced. It became a journey of uncovering what was broken, and how we might begin to repair it.

At the time, I couldn't have imagined the journey this five-year project would become, nor the incredible women whose stories it would bring it to life. The research and history in this book are essential, yes, but the personal connections—the way these inequities ripple through lives, families, and communities in the day-to-day—were just as important to bring to the surface. Through my family, my work at the center, and the connections I made, I found the voices that breathe life into this book and the people who believe, as I do, in the transformative power of storytelling to inspire change.

Marielis Rosa was one of the first people I met at the center. A brilliant first-generation Dominican American college student, she worked as my research assistant. Our conversations often went beyond data and literature reviews, touching on her experiences navigating remote learning from an overcrowded Section 8 apartment during the pandemic. Her story became one of the core narratives of this book. Today, Marielis has blossomed. After graduating from Boston University and spending a year working at an investment company, she's now pursuing her law degree at Harvard Law School. Her story of navigating systemic barriers individually to advocating for others systemically captures the essence of what this book seeks to convey.

Dorothy Oliver's name came up during a conversation with Rachael DeCruz, the center's associate director of advocacy, who codirected a short film documentary about Dorothy's efforts to protect her rural Alabama community during COVID. Watching Dorothy's story unfold on-screen moved me deeply. After interviewing her via Zoom, I had the opportunity to meet her in person in 2022 and learn more about her local leadership in her rural community. Today, Dorothy remains a steadfast advocate, rallying resources and support for her neighbors. Her work reminds us all of the power of community-driven solutions and the enduring strength of grassroots advocacy.

Through Victor Jose Santana, an antiracism trainer our team hired, I was introduced to Rosa Tupina Yaotonalcuauhtli, his godmother. Abuela Tupina embodies the intersection of cultural preservation and health. Her clinical practice, rooted in culturally sensitive therapies and traditional healing, shows how mental health care can embrace both science and heritage to foster well-being. She continues to lead La Danza annually, weaving rituals that strengthen existing community bonds and form new ones. Meeting Abuela Tupina in person and experiencing La Danza was unforgettable. Her calm wisdom, rooted in her role as an elder, and the warmth and openness of the dancers and supporters beneath the vast Texas sky created a profound sense of connection, grounding us in the rhythm of nature, as if the land itself was part of the sacred dance. The experience was one of the most transformative of my life, leaving me with a renewed appreciation for community, nature, and spiritualty.

As for me, my journey continues, shaped by the lessons and stories that fill these pages. I remain deeply committed to collaborating with others to create a healthier, more equitable world through research, teaching, and service. I have taught thousands of students across Boston University and Harvard to date, each one contributing to the ongoing conversation and work surrounding social determinants of health in their own way. And I still teach the physician students in Harvard's MHCM program, though let's just say I'm no longer the youngest person in the room nowadays.

I've also come to realize that this work is as much about listening as it is about doing. It's about meeting people where they are, hearing their lived experiences, and finding ways to collaborate across fields and communities. Each time I meet a new person or step into a room, I remind myself: the ripple effect starts here. I firmly believe that everyone—no matter their field of work, background, or expertise—has a role to play in improving the conditions around us.

Working at the center deepened my understanding of the power of narrative in doing this work. Stories connect people across divides of experience, geography, and identity. They make complex histories and data accessible, relatable, and actionable. These narratives remind us that behind every data point is a life, and that real solutions arise from understanding the systems that shape those lives.

What surprised me about writing this book was how painful it was to unlearn how to write scientifically—stripping away the jargon, the formal scholarly tone, the careful hedging that academia instills in you. Narrative writing was a completely different muscle, one I hadn't flexed in years. It meant discovering ways to bring a story to life, to write in a way that connects with the heart as much as the mind.

Despite the discomforts of a new learning curve, I found myself falling in love with the creative process. I found joy in crafting scenes that breathe, characters that feel, and moments that linger long after a page is turned. Writing this book pushed me to see the world not just through data points and research findings, but through the texture of lived experiences. It reminded me that while research has the power to inform, stories have the power to move and ultimately drive change.

Beyond the technical challenges, writing this book was emotionally exhausting. The topics, research, and stories in this book—particularly my own—are undeniably heavy and at times devastating, making it hard not to feel defeated. Yet along the way, I also found how much joy and light surround us when we make it a practice to truly look. Writing the solutions-oriented sections and staying connected with the women I interviewed gave me the hope and fuel to keep going. Inspired by La Danza, I've embraced a dual perspective: when faced with darkness, observe it without absorbing it; when you see light, lean in deeply and share it widely.

The stories of Marielis, Dorothy, and Abuela Tupina are not just theirs—they are ours. They reflect the challenges faced by millions and the possibilities that arise when we confront those challenges together. Sharing these narratives is more than an act of storytelling—it is an act of solidarity, an invitation to reimagine what is possible when we move upstream together.

As I reflect on my writing journey, I am reminded of how it began: a simple question posed in a moment of urgency. "How about a book?" It was an invitation to weave everything I had learned, through research, teaching, practice, and the stories of the people I met, into a broader narrative that might spark action.

The people in this book and many others have taught me that the fight for public health and health equity is deeply personal, profoundly collective, and entirely possible. The work doesn't end here. Sharing these stories is only the beginning. Real change happens when we carry them forward and let them shape our conversations and guide our actions. Small steps, repeated over time, can lead to extraordinary change. It only takes one person to start a ripple. It takes all of us to create a wave.

Let's dive in.

Acknowledgments

The five-year journey of developing *The Collective Cure* has been filled with moments of excitement, surprise, discomfort, growth, heartbreak, and profound joy. Writing this book has stretched me in ways I never imagined, from moments of deep self-doubt to bursts of creative clarity. It would not have been possible without the support, guidance, and inspiration from many individuals and communities. To all who contributed, directly or indirectly, to the creation of *The Collective Cure*, I am deeply grateful.

First and foremost, to my family: Luke, Ivy, and Jade—my number one fans. Your spontaneous hugs, daily humor, and belief in me (even when I was behaving like a "Treacherous Grump Grump") helped me keep going. How lucky I am to have you in my life. To my parents, thank you for instilling in me the meaning of hard work and integrity. To my mother-in-law, Reese, and my late father-in-law, Mitch, your support and wisdom continue to be gifts that I treasure.

To Marielis, Dorothy, and Abuela Tupina, your stories form the heartbeat of this book. Thank you for trusting me to tell them. You are each proof that truth is often more extraordinary than fiction.

To my dear friends, colleagues, and community who cheered me on with emoji-laden texts, memes, and GIFs—thank you for reminding me to celebrate the writing milestones, however small, along the way. Special thanks to Lisa, who joined me in experiencing La Danza.

To my agent, Ayesha Pande, my editor, Haley Lynch, and to the entire Beacon Press team: your faith in the urgency of *The Collective Cure* made this book real. Much gratitude to Teddy Turner for your sharp eye and detailed copyedits and to Susan Lumenello, managing editor, for your steady guidance and support throughout the publishing process. To my writing coach E. J. Graff, you helped me painfully and painstakingly unlearn scientific jargon and showed me how freeing (and occasionally nerve-racking) it can be to let my own voice and stories shine on the page.

To Ibram, thank you for sparking the idea for this book and showing me how words can move mountains. Your early confidence in this project was the nudge I needed to take a leap of faith and start typing.

To my colleagues in advocacy and public service, thank you for all that you do and for reminding us of the incredible power and expertise within communities. Victor Jose, your invaluable insights into Indigenous history and context enriched La Danza, providing depth and authenticity that made the experience even more meaningful. Rachael, your leadership and focus on organizing, storytelling, and filmmaking for justice have been instrumental in driving meaningful change. How proud I am to know you both.

To my research team Selenne Alatorre, Aviva Schwarz, Chas Walker, Chloe Miller, Alexandra Doegbe, and the many other research assistants who supported this project, thank you for your meticulous efforts in assisting with literature searches that kept the scholarly foundation of this book rock-solid.

To my public health professors, Drs. Ichiro Kawachi, David Williams, Nancy Krieger, and countless others, your groundbreaking work laid the foundation for so many of the themes and concepts in *The Collective Cure*.

To those who mentored and supported me along the way, Drs. Nancy Kane, Marie McCormick, S. Bryn Austin, Karen Peterson, Milagros Rosal, Stephenie Lemon, Sherry Pagoto, Laurie Pascal, Sandro Galea, Catharine Wang (no relation, but definitely a kindred spirit!), Michael McClean, the late Rich Saitz, Lois McCloskey, Carlos Rodriguez-Diaz, and more: thank you for shaping my career and my sense of purpose. You have all guided me through professional and personal challenges, advocating for me when I wasn't in the room. You showed me that life as a scholar can be rigorous *and* joyous. Special thanks to Sandro and Sherry, whose encouragement to engage the public on these issues fueled my passion for public scholarship and science communication as a form of meaningful advocacy.

To my brilliant colleagues in public health and health care, thank you for championing bold thinking and for pushing the boundaries of how we can improve lives. To the METCO staff and students, your welcoming inclusion shaped my path as well as my purpose.

To the physician and MPH students at Harvard, the undergraduate and graduate students at Boston University, and every learner I've worked with across academic halls, health care institutions, and companies: thank you for keeping me on my toes with your questions, your innovative ideas, and your determination to challenge the status quo. Seeing each of you as leaders and changemakers both inside and outside the classroom is one of the greatest joys of my career.

Finally, to you, the reader: thank *you*. I imagine you sitting with this book, perhaps curled in a comfy chair, reflecting on the stories in these pages. My hope is that *The Collective Cure* sparks new ways of thinking and talking about health—both personal and societal—and inspires you to take that next step, wherever you are, to create a more just and healthier world.

Notes

CHAPTER ONE: THE MYTH OF THE GREAT EQUALIZER

1. Marielis Rosa, interview by Monica Wang, Boston, MA, Mar. 2, 2022.

2. David Cutler and Adriana Lleras-Muney, "Education and Health: Evaluating Theories and Evidence," *Making Americans Healthier: Social and Economic Policy as Health Policy* (2006): 12352, doi: 10.3386/w12352; Damon Clark and Heather Royer, "The Effect of Education on Adult Mortality and Health: Evidence from Britain," *American Economic Review* 103, no. 6 (2013): 2087–2120, doi: 10.1257/aer.103.6.2087.

3. US Social Security Administration, "Education and Lifetime Earnings," Nov. 2015, https://www.ssa.gov/policy/docs/research-summaries/education-earnings.html.

4. US Bureau of Labor Statistics, "Learn More, Earn More: Education Leads to Higher Wages, Lower Unemployment," May 2020, https://www.bls.gov/careeroutlook/2020/data-on-display/education-pays.htm.

5. David P. Baker, *The Schooled Society: The Educational Transformation of Global Culture* (Stanford, CA: Stanford University Press, 2014).

6. Charles W. Mueller and Toby L. Parcel, "Measures of Socioeconomic Status: Alternatives and Recommendations," *Child Development* 52 (1981): 13–30, doi: 10.2307/1129211.

7. M. Maria Glymour, Mauricio Avendano, and Ichiro Kawachi, "Socioeconomic Status and Health," in *Social Epidemiology*, 2nd ed., online ed., ed. Lisa F. Berkman, Ichiro Kawachi, and M. Maria Glymour (New York: Oxford Academic, 2015).

8. Fjolla Kondirolli and Naveen Sunder, "Mental Health Effects of Education," *Health Economics* 31, Suppl. 2 (2022): 22–39, doi: 10.1002/hec.4565.

9. Giorgio Brunello et al., "The Causal Effect of Education on Health: What Is the Role of Health Behaviors?" *Health Economics* 25, no. 3 (2016): 314–36, doi: 10.1002/hec.3141.

10. Iris Van der Heide et al., "The Relationship Between Health, Education, and Health Literacy: Results from the Dutch Adult Literacy and Life Skills Survey," *Journal of Health Communication* 18, Suppl. 1 (2013): 172–184, doi: 10.1080/10810730.2013.825668.

11. William Evans, Barbara Wolfe, and Nancy Adler, "The SES and Health Gradient: A Brief Review of the Literature" (2012): 1–37; Nancy E. Adler et al.,

"Socioeconomic Status and Health: The Challenge of the Gradient," *American Psychologist* 49, no. 1 (1994): 15–24, doi: 10.1037//0003-066x.49.1.15.

12. A. Espelt et al., "Socioeconomic Position and Type 2 Diabetes Mellitus in Europe 1999–2009: A Panorama of Inequalities," *Current Diabetes Review* 7 (2011): 148–58, doi: 10.2174/157339911795843131; Benjamin D. Bray et al. and SSNAP Collaboration, "Socioeconomic Disparities in First Stroke Incidence, Quality of Care, and Survival: A Nationwide Registry-Based Cohort Study of 44 Million Adults in England," *Lancet Public Health* 3 (2018): e185–e193, doi: 10.1016/S2468-2667(18)30030-6.

13. Simon Condliffe and Charles R. Link, "The Relationship Between Economic Status and Child Health: Evidence from the United States," *American Economic Review* 98, no. 4 (2008): 1605–18, doi: 10.1257/aer.98.4.1605; Anne Case, Darren Lubotsky, and Christina Paxson, "Economic Status and Health in Childhood: The Origins of the Gradient," *American Economic Review* 92, no. 5 (2002): 1308–34.

14. Marialaura Bonaccio et al., "Interaction Between Education and Income on the Risk of All-Cause Mortality: Prospective Results from the MOLI-SANI Study," *International Journal of Public Health* 61 (2016): 765–76, doi: 10.1007/s00038-016-0822-z.

15. Silvia Stringhini et al. and the LIFEPATH Consortium, "Socioeconomic Status and the 25×25 Risk Factors as Determinants of Premature Mortality: A Multicohort Study and Meta-Analysis of 1.7 Million Men and Women," *Lancet* 389, no. 10075 (2017): 1229–37, doi: 10.1016/S0140-6736(16)32380-7.

16. James Banks et al., "Disease and Disadvantage in the United States and in England," *JAMA* 295, no. 17 (2006): 2037–45, doi: 10.1001/jama.295.17.2037.

17. Paula Braveman and Laura Gottlieb, "The Social Determinants of Health: It's Time to Consider the Causes of the Causes," *Public Health Reports* 129, Suppl. 2 (2014): 19–31, doi: 10.1177/00333549141291S206; World Health Organization, "Social Determinants of Health," 2024, https://www.who.int/health-topics/social-determinants-of-health.

18. Joia Crear-Perry et al., "Social and Structural Determinants of Health Inequities in Maternal Health," *Journal of Women's Health* 30, no. 2 (2021): 230–35, doi: 10.1089/jwh.2020.8882.

19. Susan Dynarski and Judith Scott-Clayton, "Financial Aid Policy: Lessons from Research," *Future Child* 23, no. 1 (2013): 67–91, doi: 10.1353/foc.2013.0002; Michael B. Paulsen et al., "Going to College: How Social, Economic, and Educational Factors Influence the Decisions Students Make," *Journal of Higher Education* 72 (2001): 383, doi: 10.2307/2649342.

20. Sean F. Reardon, "The Widening Academic Achievement Gap Between the Rich and the Poor: New Evidence and Possible Explanations," in *Whither Opportunity*, ed. G. J. Duncan and R. J. Murnane (New York: Russell Sage, 2011), 91–116; Russell W. Rumberger and Gregory J. Palardy, "Does Segregation Still Matter? The Impact of Student Composition on Academic Achievement in High School," *Teachers College Record* 107, no. 9 (2005): 1999–2045, doi: 10.1111/j.1467-9620.2005.00583.x.

21. Taylor Odle, Jennifer A. Delaney, and Preston Magouirk, "Complex Applications Create Barriers to College—Some Are Trying to Change That,"

Brookings Institute, Oct. 23, 2023, https://www.brookings.edu/articles/complex-applications-create-barriers-to-college-some-are-trying-to-change-that/.

22. Emma García and Elaine Weiss, "Education Inequalities at the School Starting Gate: Gaps, Trends, and Strategies to Address Them," Economic Policy Institute, Sept. 27, 2017, https://www.epi.org/publication/education-inequalities-at-the-school-starting-gate/.

23. Ichiro Kawachi, Norman Daniels, and Dean E. Robinson, "Health Disparities by Race and Class: Why Both Matter," *Health Affairs* 24, no. 2 (2005): 343–52, doi: 10.1377/hlthaff.24.2.343; David R. Williams et al., "Race, Socioeconomic Status, and Health: Complexities, Ongoing Challenges, and Research Opportunities," *Annals of the New York Academy of Sciences* 1186 (2010): 69–101, doi: 10.1111/j.1749-6632.2009.05339.x.

24. Samuel H. Fishman et al., "Race/Ethnicity, Maternal Educational Attainment, and Infant Mortality in the United States," *Biodemography and Social Biology* 66, no. 1 (2020): 1–26, doi: 10.1080/19485565.2020.1793659.

25. C. Andre Christie-Mizell, "Neighborhood Disadvantage and Poor Health: The Consequences of Race, Gender, and Age Among Young Adults," *International Journal of Environmental Research and Public Health* 19, no. 13 (2022): 8107, doi: 10.3390/ijerph19138107; Catherine E. Ross and John Mirowsky, "Neighborhood Disadvantage, Disorder, and Health," *Journal of Health and Social Behavior* 42, no. 3 (2001): 258–76, PMID: 11668773, doi: 10.2307/3090214.

26. Kathleen T. Call et al., "Barriers to Care in an Ethnically Diverse Publicly Insured Population: Is Health Care Reform Enough?" *Medical Care* 52, no. 8 (2014): 720–27, doi: 10.1097/MLR.0000000000000172; N. Douthit et al., "Exposing Some Important Barriers to Health Care Access in the Rural USA," *Public Health* 129, no. 6 (2015): 611–20, doi: 10.1016/j.puhe.2015.04.001.

27. Robert A. Hummer and Elaine M. Hernandez, "The Effect of Educational Attainment on Adult Mortality in the United States," *Population Bulletin* 68, no. 1 (2013): 1–16.

28. Brian L. Rostron, John L. Boies, and Elizabeth Arias, "Education Reporting and Classification on Death Certificates in the United States," *Vital and Health Statistics* 2, no. 151 (2010): 1–21.

29. Angela D'Adamo et al., "Health Disparities in Past Influenza Pandemics: A Scoping Review of the Literature," *Social Science Medicine Population Health* 21 (2023): 101314, doi: 10.1016/j.ssmph.2023.101516.

30. Monica L. Wang, "What Is Driving Racial/Ethnic Disparities in COVID-19 Morbidity and Mortality?" *Medium*, Apr. 12, 2020, https://medium.com/age-of-awareness/what-is-driving-racial-ethnic-disparities-in-covid-19-morbidity-and-mortality-49f31cbcdd3a.

31. National Academies of Sciences, Engineering, and Medicine, *Integrating Social Care into the Delivery of Health Care: Moving Upstream to Improve the Nation's Health* (Washington, DC: National Academies Press, 2019).

32. John B. McKinlay, "A Case of Refocusing Upstream: The Political Economy of Illness," in *Patients, Physicians, and Illness: A Sourcebook in Behavioral Science and Health*, 3rd ed., ed. E. G. Jaco (London: The Free Press, 1979), 9–25.

33. David R. Williams et al., "Moving Upstream: How Interventions That Address the Social Determinants of Health Can Improve Health and Reduce

Disparities," *Journal of Public Health Management and Practice* 14, Suppl. (2008): S8–S17, doi: 10.1097/01.PHH.0000338382.36695.42.

34. C. J. Avila and A. B. Frakt, "Raising the Minimum Wage and Public Health," *JAMA Health Forum* 4, no. 2 (Jan. 2021): e201587, doi: 10.1001/jama healthforum.2020.1587.

35. B. D. Sommers, K. Baicker, and A. M. Epstein, "Mortality and Access to Care Among Adults After State Medicaid Expansions," *New England Journal of Medicine* 13, no. 367 (Sept. 2012): 1025–34, doi: 10.1056/NEJMsa1202099.

36. Lawrence Schweinhart and David Weikart, *The High/Scope Perry Preschool Program*, Primary Prevention Works, doi: 10.1037/10064-005; Frances A. Campbell et al., "Adult Outcomes as a Function of an Early Childhood Educational Program: An Abecedarian Project Follow-Up," *Developmental Psychology* 48, no. 4 (July 2012): 1033–43, doi: 10.1037/a0026644; Frances A. Campbell and Craig T. Ramey, "Effects of Early Intervention on Intellectual and Academic Achievement: A Follow-Up Study of Children from Low-Income Families," *Child Development* 65, no. 2 (Apr. 1994): 684–98, doi: 10.1111/j.1467-8624.1994.tb00773.x.

37. M. Y. Yen et al., "From SARS in 2003 to H1N1 in 2009: Lessons Learned from Taiwan in Preparation for the Next Pandemic," *Journal of Hospital Infection* 87, no. 4 (2014): 185–93, doi: 10.1016/j.jhin.2014.05.005; Shikha Kukreti et al., "Response to the COVID-19 Pandemic in Taiwan," in *Global Perspectives of COVID-19 Pandemic on Health, Education, and Role of Media*, ed. S. Pachauri and A. Pachauri (Singapore: Springer, 2023).

38. Suetgiin Soon, Chelsea C. Chou, and Shih-Jiunn Shi, "Withstanding the Plague: Institutional Resilience of the East Asian Welfare State," *Social Policy and Administration* 55, no. 2 (2021): 374–87, doi: 10.1111/spol.12713; Jun Jie Woo, "Singapore's Social Policy Response to Covid-19: Focusing on Jobs and Employment," *CRC 1342, Covid-19 Social Policy Response Series 16/2021*, Bremen, 2021, https://www.socialpolicydynamics.de/f/9678d75f10.pdf.

39. W. C. Lee and C. Y. Ong, "Overview of Rapid Mitigating Strategies in Singapore During the COVID-19 Pandemic," *Public Health* 185 (2020): 15–17, doi: 10.1016/j.puhe.2020.05.015.

40. Gabriel Hoh et al., "Factors Influencing Asia-Pacific Countries' Success Level in Curbing COVID-19: A Review Using a Social-Ecological System (SES) Framework," *International Journal of Environmental Research and Public Health* 18, no. 4 (2021): 1704, doi: 10.3390/ijerph18041704.

41. Pan Suk Kim, "South Korea's Fast Response to Coronavirus Disease: Implications on Public Policy and Public Management Theory," *Public Management Review* 23, no. 12 (2021): 1736–47, doi: 10.1080/14719037.2020.1766266; Alvin Qijia et al., "Health System Resilience in Managing the COVID-19 Pandemic: Lessons from Singapore," *BMJ Global Health* 5, no. 9 (2020): e003317, doi: 10.1136/bmjgh-2020-003317.

CHAPTER TWO: THE SPACES IN BETWEEN

1. US Census Bureau, "Improved Race and Ethnicity Measures Reveal United States Population Much More Multiracial," Aug. 2021, https://www.census.gov /library/stories/2021/08/improved-race-ethnicity-measures-reveal-united-states -population-much-more-multiracial.html.

2. Stephen Cornell and Douglas Hartmann, *Ethnicity and Race: Making Identities in a Changing World* (Thousand Oaks, CA: Pine Forge Press, 1998).

3. Michael Omi and Howard Winant, *Racial Formation in the United States: From the 1960s to the 1990s*, 3rd ed. (New York: Routledge, 1994).

4. National Research Council (US) Panel on Race, Ethnicity, and Health in Later Life, *Critical Perspectives on Racial and Ethnic Differences in Health in Late Life*, ed. N. B. Anderson, R. A. Bulatao, and B. Cohen (Washington, DC: National Academies Press, 2004), chapter 2, "Racial and Ethnic Identification, Official Classifications, and Health Disparities," https://www.ncbi.nlm.nih.gov/books/NBK25522/.

5. Raj Bhopal, "Glossary of Terms Relating to Ethnicity and Race: For Reflection and Debate," *Journal of Epidemiology and Community Health* 58, no. 6 (2004): 441–45, doi: 10.1136/jech.2003.013466.

6. National Museum of African American History and Culture, "Historical Foundations of Race," Smithsonian Institution, https://nmaahc.si.edu/learn/talking-about-race/topics/historical-foundations-race.

7. Ivan Hannaford, *Race: The History of an Idea in the West* (Baltimore: Johns Hopkins University Press, 1996).

8. Jane H. Yamashiro, "The Social Construction of Race and Minorities in Japan," *Sociology Compass* 7, no. 2 (2013): 147–61, doi: 10.1111/soc4.12013.

9. Peggy A. Lovell, "Development and the Persistence of Racial Inequality in Brazil: 1950–1991," *Journal of Development Areas* 33 (1999): 395–418.

10. Michel Agier, "Racism, Culture and Black Identity in Brazil," *Bulletin of Latin American Research* 14 (1995): 245–64, doi: 10.1111/j.1470-9856.1995.tb00010.x.

11. Stanley R. Bailey, Mara Loveman, and Jeronimo O. Muniz, "Measures of 'Race' and the Analysis of Racial Inequality in Brazil," *Social Science Research* 42, no. 1 (2013): 106–19, doi: 10.1016/j.ssresearch.2012.06.006.

12. Heidi L. Lujan and Stephen E. DiCarlo, "The Racist 'One Drop Rule' Influencing Science: It Is Time to Stop Teaching 'Race Corrections' in Medicine," *Advances in Physiology Education* 45, no. 3 (2021): 644–50, doi: 10.1152/advan.00063.2021.

13. "One Drop Rule," *Encyclopedia of Arkansas*, https://encyclopediaofarkansas.net/entries/one-drop-rule-5365/.

14. F. James Davis, *Who Is Black? One Nation's Definition* (University Park: Pennsylvania State University Press, 1991).

15. Stephanie Yom and Maichu Lor, "Advancing Health Disparities Research: The Need to Include Asian American Subgroup Populations," *Journal of Racial and Ethnic Health Disparities* 9, no. 6 (2022): 2248–82, doi: 10.1007/s40615-021-01164-8.

16. Ryan F. Lei and Galen V. Bodenhausen, "Racial Assumptions Color the Mental Representation of Social Class," *Frontiers in Psychology* 8 (2017): 519, doi: 10.3389/fpsyg.2017.00519.

17. Riley Whiting and Suzanne Bartle-Haring, "Variations in the Association Between Education and Self-Reported Health by Race/Ethnicity and Structural Racism," *Social Science Medicine Population Health* 19 (2022): 101136, doi: 10.1016/j.ssmph.2022.101136.

18. National Academies of Sciences, Engineering, and Medicine, Health and Medicine Division, Board on Population Health and Public Health Practice, Committee on Community-Based Solutions to Promote Health Equity in the United States, *Communities in Action: Pathways to Health Equity*, ed. A. Baciu, Y. Negussie, A. Geller, et al. (Washington, DC: National Academies Press, 2017), chapter 2, "The State of Health Disparities in the United States."

19. Richard Cooper et al., "An International Comparative Study of Blood Pressure in Populations of European vs. African Descent," *BMC Medicine* 3 (2005): 2, doi: 10.1186/1741-7015-3-2.

20. *Nature Genetics*, "Genetics for the Human Race," Supplemental, Oct. 26, 2004, https://www.nature.com/collections/cpzwxlgvzj.

21. Camara P. Jones, "Levels of Racism: A Theoretic Framework and a Gardener's Tale," *American Journal of Public Health* 90, no. 8 (2000): 1212–15.

22. Alexander R. Green et al., "Implicit Bias Among Physicians and Its Prediction of Thrombolysis Decisions for Black and White Patients," *Journal of General Internal Medicine* 22, no. 9 (2007): 1231–38, doi: 10.1007/s11606-007-0258-5.

23. William J. Hall et al., "Implicit Racial/Ethnic Bias Among Health Care Professionals and Its Influence on Health Care Outcomes: A Systematic Review," *American Journal of Public Health* 105, no. 12 (2015): e60–e76, doi: 10.2105/AJPH .2015.302903.

24. Ronald Wyatt, "Pain and Ethnicity," *AMA Journal of Ethics* 15, no. 5 (2013): 449–54, doi: 10.1001/virtualmentor.2013.15.5.pfor1-1305; Kelly M. Hoffman et al., "Racial Bias in Pain Assessment and Treatment Recommendations, and False Beliefs About Biological Differences Between Blacks and Whites," *Proceedings of the National Academy of Sciences* 113, no. 16 (2016): 4296–4301, doi: 10.1073 /pnas.1516047113; Monica L. Wang and Olivia Jacobs, "From Awareness to Action: Pathways to Equity in Pain Management," *Health Equity* 7, no. 1 (2023): 416–18, doi: 10.1089/heq.2023.0179.

25. Amal N. Trivedi and John Z. Ayanian, "Perceived Discrimination and Use of Preventive Health Services," *Journal of General Internal Medicine* 21, no. 6 (2006): 553–58, doi: 10.1111/j.1525-1497.2006.00413.x.

26. David R. Williams, "Stress and the Mental Health of Populations of Color: Advancing Our Understanding of Race-Related Stressors," *Journal of Health and Social Behavior* 59, no. 4 (2018): 466–85, doi: 10.1177/0022146518814251; Monica L. Wang and Marie-Rachelle Narcisse, "Discrimination, Depression, and Anxiety Among US Adults," *JAMA Network Open* 8, no. 3 (2025): e252404, doi: 10.1001 /jamanetworkopen.2025.2404.

27. Tené T. Lewis, Courtney D. Cogburn, and David R. Williams, "Self-Reported Experiences of Discrimination and Health: Scientific Advances, Ongoing Controversies, and Emerging Issues," *Annual Review of Clinical Psychology* 11 (2015): 407–40, doi: 10.1146/annurev-clinpsy-032814-112728; Yin Paradies et al., "Racism as a Determinant of Health: A Systematic Review and Meta-Analysis," *PLOS ONE* 10, no. 9 (2015): e0138511, doi: 10.1371/journal.pone.0138511.

28. David R. Williams and Selina A. Mohammed, "Discrimination and Racial Disparities in Health: Evidence and Needed Research," *Journal of Behavioral Medicine* 32, no. 1 (2009): 20–47, doi: 10.1007/s10865-008-9185-0.

29. Arline T. Geronimus, "The Weathering Hypothesis and the Health of African-American Women and Infants: Evidence and Speculations," *Ethnicity and Disease* 2 (1992): 207–21; Arline T. Geronimus et al., "'Weathering' and Age Patterns of Allostatic Load Scores Among Blacks and Whites in the United States," *American Journal of Public Health* 96, no. 5 (2006): 826–33, doi: 10.2105/AJPH .2004.060749.

30. O. Kenrik Duru et al., "Allostatic Load Burden and Racial Disparities in Mortality," *Journal of the National Medical Association* 104, nos. 1–2 (2012): 89–95, doi: 10.1016/s0027-9684(15)30120-6.

31. David H. Chae et al., "Racial Discrimination and Telomere Shortening Among African Americans: The Coronary Artery Risk Development in Young Adults (CARDIA) Study," *Health Psychology* 39, no. 3 (2020): 209–19; Elizabeth J. Pantesco et al., "Multiple Forms of Discrimination, Social Status, and Telomere Length: Interactions Within Race," *Psychoneuroendocrinology* 98 (2018): 119–26, doi: 10.1016/j.psyneuen.2018.08.012.

32. Darlene Powell-Hopson and Derek S. Hopson, "Implications of Doll Color Preferences Among Black Preschool Children and White Preschool Children," *Journal of Black Psychology* 14, no. 2 (1988): 57–63, doi: 10.1177/00957984 880142004.

33. Claude M. Steele, "A Threat in the Air: How Stereotypes Shape Intellectual Identity and Performance," *American Psychologist* 52, no. 6 (1997): 613–29, doi: 10.1037//0003-066x.52.6.613.

34. Claude S. Fischer, Michael Hout, Martín Sánchez Jankowski, Samuel R. Lucas, Ann Swidler, and Kim Voss, *Inequality by Design: Cracking the Bell Curve Myth* (Princeton, NJ: Princeton University Press, 1996).

35. Jim Blascovitch et al., "African Americans and High Blood Pressure: The Role of Stereotype Threat," *Psychological Science* 12, no. 3 (2001): 225–29, doi: 10.1111/1467-9280.00340.

36. Marc A. Zimmerman et al., "Youth Empowerment Solutions: Evaluation of an After-School Program to Engage Middle School Students in Community Change," *Health Education and Behavior* 45, no. 1 (2018): 20–31, doi: 10.1177/1090198117710491.

37. Linda S. Sprague Martinez et al., "Critical Discourse, Applied Inquiry, and Public Health Action with Urban Middle School Students: Lessons Learned Engaging Youth in Critical Service-Learning," *Journal of Community Practice* 25, no. 1 (2017): 68–89, doi: 10.1080/10705422.2016.1269251; Beti Thompson et al., "Strategies to Empower Communities to Reduce Health Disparities," *Health Affairs* 35, no. 8 (2016): 1424–28, doi: 10.1377/hlthaff.2015.1364.

38. Jaqueline Hoying and Bernadette M. Melnyk, "COPE: A Pilot Study With Urban-Dwelling Minority Sixth-Grade Youth to Improve Physical Activity and Mental Health Outcomes," *Journal of School Nursing* 32, no. 5 (2016): 347–56, doi: 10.1177/1059840516635.

39. Jeffrey S. Geller et al., "Pediatric Obesity Empowerment Model Group Medical Visits (POEM-GMV) as Treatment for Pediatric Obesity in an Underserved Community," *Child Obesity* 11, no. 5 (2015): 638–46, doi.org/10.1089/chi .2014.0163.

40. Stephanie Rushing et al., "Healthy & Empowered Youth: A Positive Youth Development Program for Native Youth," *American Journal of Preventive Medicine* 52, no. 3S3 (2017): S263–S267, doi: 10.1016/j.amepre.2016.10.024.

41. Bernadette Mazurek Melnyk et al., "Twelve-Month Effects of the COPE Healthy Lifestyles TEEN Program on Overweight and Depressive Symptoms in High School Adolescents," *Journal of School Health* 85, no. 12 (2015): 861–70, doi: 10.1111/josh.12342.

42. Geoffrey L. Cohen and David K. Sherman, "The Psychology of Change: Self-Affirmation and Social Psychological Intervention," *Annual Review of Psychology* 65 (2014): 222–71, doi: 10.1146/annurev-psych-010213-115137.

43. Mandy Truong, Yin Paradies, and Naomi Priest, "Interventions to Improve Cultural Competency in Healthcare: A Systematic Review of Reviews," *BMC Health Services Research* 14 (2014): 99, doi: 10.1186/1472-6963-14-99.

44. Patricia G. Devine et al., "Long-Term Reduction in Implicit Race Bias: A Prejudice Habit-Breaking Intervention," *Journal of Experimental Social Psychology* 48 (2012): 1267–78, doi: 10.1016/j.jesp.2012.06.003.

45. Ivy W. Maina et al., "A Decade of Studying Implicit Racial/Ethnic Bias in Healthcare Providers Using the Implicit Association Test," *Social Science and Medicine* 199 (2018): 219–29, doi: 10.1016/j.socscimed.2017.05.009.

46. Monica L. Wang et al., "A Systematic Review of Diversity, Equity, and Inclusion and Antiracism Training Studies: Findings and Future Directions," *Translational Behavioral Medicine* 14, no. 3 (2024): 156–71, doi: 10.1093/tbm/ibado61.

47. Victoria Haldane et al., "Community Participation in Health Services Development, Implementation, and Evaluation: A Systematic Review of Empowerment, Health, Community, and Process Outcomes," *PLoS One* 14 (2019): e0226970, doi: 10.1371/journal.pone.0216112.

CHAPTER THREE: A TALE OF TWO NEIGHBORHOODS

1. Dolores Acevedo-Garcia et al., "What's New in the Child Opportunity Index 3.0?" *Diversity Data Kids*, Mar. 4, 2024, https://www.diversitydatakids.org/research-library/blog/whats-new-child-opportunity-index-30.

2. "The New Deal," History.com, Mar. 29, 2021, https://www.history.com/topics/great-depression/new-deal.

3. Richard Rothstein, *The Color of Law: A Forgotten History of How Our Government Segregated America* (New York: Liveright, 2018); Amy E. Hillier, "Residential Security Maps and Neighborhood Appraisals: The Home Owners' Loan Corporation and the Case of Philadelphia," *Social Science History* 29 (2005): 207–33.

4. Amy E. Hillier, "Redlining and the Home Owners' Loan Corporation," *Journal of Urban History* 29 (2003): 394–420.

5. Jacob W. Faber, "We Built This: Consequences of New Deal Era Intervention in America's Racial Geography," *American Sociological Review* 85, no. 5 (2020): 739–75, doi: 10.1177/0003122420948464.

6. Price Fishback et al., "New Evidence on Redlining by Federal Housing Programs in the 1930s," *Journal of Urban Economics* 141 (2024): 103462, doi: 10.1016/j.jue.2022.103462.

7. Camara P. Jones, "Levels of Racism: A Theoretic Framework and a Gardener's Tale," *American Journal of Public Health* 90, no. 8 (2000): 1212–15, doi: 10.2105/ajph.90.8.1212.

8. Nancy Krieger, "Discrimination and Health Inequities," *International Journal of Health Services* 44, no. 4 (2014): 643–710, doi: 10.2190/HS.44.4.b.

9. Mehrsa Baradaran, *The Color of Money: Black Banks and the Racial Wealth Gap* (Cambridge, MA: Harvard University Press, 2017).

10. Na Zhao, "Homeownership Rates by Race and Ethnicity," *Eye on Housing*, Feb. 2024, https://eyeonhousing.org/2024/02/homeownership-rates-by-race-and -ethnicity-3/.

11. Isabela Espadas Barros Leal, "A $1 Million Wealth Gap Now Divides White Families from Black and Hispanic Ones, Research Shows," NBC News, Apr. 25, 2024, https://www.nbcnews.com/news/latino/1-million-wealth-gap-white -black-hispanic-families-rcna149252.

12. Bruce D. Baker, Matthew Di Carlo, and Preston C. Green III, "Segregation and School Funding: How Housing Discrimination Reproduces Inequality," Albert Shanker Institute, May 2022, https://www.shankerinstitute.org/sites /default/files/2022-05/SEGreportfinal.pdf.

13. Lindsey Burke and Jude Schwalbach, "Housing Redlining and Its Lingering Effects on Education Opportunity," Heritage Foundation, Mar. 11, 2021, https://www.heritage.org/education/report/housing-redlining-and-its-lingering -effects-education-opportunity.

14. "Report Finds $23 Billion Racial Funding Gap for Schools," *Washington Post*, Feb. 25, 2019, https://www.washingtonpost.com/local/education/report-finds -23-billion-racial-funding-gap-for-schools/2019/02/25/d562b704-3915-11e9-a06c -3ec8ed509d15_story.html.

15. Daniel Aaronson, Daniel Hartley, and Bhashkar Mazumder, "The Effects of the 1930s HOLC 'Redlining' Maps," *American Economic Journal: Economic Policy* 13, no. 4 (2020): 355–92, doi: 10.1257/pol.20190414.

16. S. Namin et al., "The Legacy of the Home Owners' Loan Corporation and the Political Ecology of Urban Trees and Air Pollution in the United States," *Social Science & Medicine* 246 (Feb. 2020): 112758, doi: 10.1016/j.socscimed.2019 .112758.

17. Jeremy Hoffman, Vivek Shandas, and Nicholas Pendleton, "The Effects of Historical Housing Policies on Resident Exposure to Intra-Urban Heat: A Study of 108 U.S. Urban Areas," *Climate* 8, no. 1 (2020): 12, doi: 10.0.3390/cli8010012.

18. Anthony Nardone et al., "Associations Between Historical Residential Redlining and Current Age-Adjusted Rates of Emergency Department Visits Due to Asthma Across Eight Cities in California: An Ecological Study," *Lancet Planetary Health* 4, no. 1 (2020): e24–e31, doi: 10.1016/S2542-5196(19)30241-4.

19. Yasamin Shaker et al., "Redlining, Racism and Food Access in U.S. Urban Cores," *Agricultural and Human Values* 40, no. 1 (2023): 101–12, doi: 10.1007 /s10460-022-10340-3.

20. Pamela J. Trangenstein et al., "Alcohol Outlet Clusters and Population Disparities," *Journal of Urban Health* 97 (2020): 123–36, doi: 10.1007/s11524 -019-00372-2.

21. Eun Kyung Lee et al., "Health Outcomes in Redlined Versus Non-Redlined Neighborhoods: A Systematic Review and Meta-Analysis," *Social Science & Medicine* 294 (2022): 114696, doi: 10.1016/j.socscimed.2021.114696.

22. Anna W. Wright et al., "Systematic Review: Exposure to Community Violence and Physical Health Outcomes in Youth," *Journal of Pediatric Psychology* 42, no. 4 (2017): 364–78, doi: 10.1093/jpepsy/jsw088; Xi Huang, Christian King, and Jennifer McAtee, "Exposure to Violence, Neighborhood Context, and Health-Related Outcomes in Low-Income Urban Mothers," *Health & Place* 54 (2018): 138–48, doi: 10.1016/j.healthplace.2018.09.008.

23. Sara F. Jacoby et al., "The Enduring Impact of Historical and Structural Racism on Urban Violence in Philadelphia," *Social Science & Medicine* 199 (2018): 87–95, doi: 10.1016/j.socscimed.2017.05.038.

24. Jacoby et al., "The Enduring Impact of Historical and Structural Racism on Urban Violence in Philadelphia," 87–95; Matthew Benns et al., "The Impact of Historical Racism on Modern Gun Violence: Redlining in the City of Louisville, KY," *Injury* 51, no. 10 (2020): 2192–98, doi: 10.1016/j.injury.2020.06.042.

25. Richard C. Sadler et al., "Inequitable Housing Practices and Youth Internalizing Symptoms: Mediation Via Perceptions of Neighborhood Cohesion," *Urban Planning* 7, no. 4 (2022): 153–66, doi: 10.17645/up.v7i4.5410.

26. Nancy Krieger et al., "Cancer Stage at Diagnosis, Historic Redlining, and Current Neighborhood Characteristics: Breast, Cervical, and Colorectal Cancer, Massachusetts, 2001–2015," *American Journal of Public Health* (2020), doi: 10.1093/aje/kwaa045; Leonard E. Egede et al., "Modern Day Consequences of Historic Redlining: Finding a Path Forward," *Journal of General Internal Medicine* 38, no. 6 (2023): 1534–37, doi: 10.1007/s11606-023-08051-4.

27. Min Li and Faxi Yuan, "Historical Redlining and Resident Exposure to COVID-19: A Study of New York City," *Race and Social Problems* 14, no. 2 (2022): 85–100, doi: 10.1007/s12552-021-09338-z.

28. National Community Reinvestment Coalition, "Redlining and Neighborhood," https://ncrc.org/holc-health/.

29. Giovanni Appolon et al., "Association Between Redlining and Spatial Access to Pharmacies," *JAMA Network Open* 6, no. 8 (2023): e2327315, doi: 10.1001/jamanetworkopen.2023.27315; Elizabeth Eisenhauer, "In Poor Health: Supermarket Redlining and Urban Nutrition," *GeoJournal* (2001): 125–33, doi: 10.1023/A:1015772503007.

30. Hernan Galperin, Thai V. Le, and Kurt Duam, "Who Gets Access to Fast Broadband? Evidence from Los Angeles County," *Government Information Quarterly* 38, no. 3 (2021): 101594, doi: 10.1016/j.giq.2021.101594.

31. Monica L. Wang, Cristina M. Gago, and Kate Rodriguez, "Digital Redlining—The Invisible Structural Determinant of Health," *JAMA* 331, no. 15 (2024): 1267–68, doi: 10.1001/jama.2024.1628.

32. Paula A. Braveman et al., "Systemic and Structural Racism: Definitions, Examples, Health Damages, and Approaches to Dismantling," *Health Affairs* 41, no. 2 (2022): 171–78, doi: 10.1377/hlthaff.2021.01394.

33. Emilio J. Castilla, "The Resilience of Racial Inequality: The Persistence of Discrimination in the Workplace," Wharton School of the University of

Pennsylvania, 2008, https://ideas.wharton.upenn.edu/wp-content/uploads/2018/07/Castilla-2008.pdf.

34. Marianne Bertrand and Sendhil Mullainathan, "Are Emily and Greg More Employable Than Lakisha and Jamal? A Field Experiment on Labor Market Discrimination," *American Economic Review* 94, no. 4 (2004): 991–1013, doi: 10.1257/0002828042002561.

35. Patrick Kline, Evan K. Rose, and Christopher R. Walters, "Systemic Discrimination Among Large U.S. Employers," *Quarterly Journal of Economics* 137, no. 4 (Nov. 2022): 1963–2036, doi: 10.1093/qje/qjac024.

36. Travis Riddle and Stacey Sinclair, "Racial Disparities in School-Based Disciplinary Actions Are Associated with County-Level Rates of Racial Bias," *Proceedings of the National Academy of Sciences U.S.A.* 116, no. 17 (2019): 8255–60, doi: 10.1073/pnas.1808307116.

37. Young Whan Choi, "Racial Bias in Standardized Testing," *NextGen Learning*, Mar. 31, 2020, https://www.nextgenlearning.org/articles/racial-bias-standardized-testing.

38. Roby Chatterji, Neil Campbell, and Abby Quirk, "Closing Advanced Coursework Equity Gaps for All Students," Center for American Progress, June 2021, https://files.eric.ed.gov/fulltext/ED617048.pdf; Kayla Patrick, Allison Socol, and Ivy Morgan, "Inequities in Advanced Coursework: What's Driving Them and What Leaders Can Do," Education Trust, Jan. 2020, https://edtrust.org/wp-content/uploads/2014/09/Inequities-in-Advanced-Coursework-Whats-Driving-Them-and-What-Leaders-Can-Do-January-2019.pdf.

39. Rebecca C. Hetey and Jennifer L. Eberhardt, "The Numbers Don't Speak for Themselves: Racial Disparities and the Persistence of Inequality in the Criminal Justice System," *Current Directions in Psychological Science* 27, no. 3 (2018): 183–87, doi: 10.1177/0963721418763931.

40. Min Li and Faxi Yuan, "Historical Redlining and Food Environments: A Study of 102 Urban Areas in the United States," *Health Place* 75 (2022): 102775, doi: 10.1016/j.healthplace.2022.102775.

41. Anne Barnhill et al., "The Racialized Marketing of Unhealthy Foods and Beverages: Perspectives and Potential Remedies," *Journal of Law, Medicine & Ethics* 50, no. 1 (2022): 52–59, doi: 10.1017/jme.2022.8.

42. Jennifer L. Harris, "Targeted Food Marketing to Black and Hispanic Consumers: The Tobacco Playbook," *American Journal of Public Health* 110, no. 3 (2020): 271–72, doi: 10.2105/AJPH.2019.305518.

43. Jesse Cross-Call, "Medicaid Expansion Has Helped Narrow Racial Disparities in Health Coverage and Access," Center on Budget and Policy Priorities, Oct. 21, 2020, https://www.cbpp.org/research/health/medicaid-expansion-has-helped-narrow-racial-disparities-in-health-coverage-and.

44. Antwan Jones, Gregory D. Squires, and Carolynn Nixon, "Ecological Associations Between Inclusionary Zoning Policies and Cardiovascular Disease Risk Prevalence: An Observational Study," *Circulation: Cardiovascular Quality and Outcomes* 14, no. 9 (2021): e007807, doi: 10.1161/CIRCOUTCOMES.120.007807.

45. Federal Communications Commission, "Affordable Connectivity Program," https://www.fcc.gov/acp.

46. City of Charlotte, "City Seeks to Close Digital Divide Through Access Charlotte," June 21, 2023, https://www.charlottenc.gov/CS-Prep/City-News /City-of-Charlotte-Seeks-to-Close-Digital-Divide-through-Access-Charlotte.

47. National League of Cities, "Investing in Digital Equity Solutions: Infrastructure," *Digital Equity Playbook: How City Leaders Can Bridge the Digital Divide*, Dec. 9, 2021, https://www.nlc.org/resource/digital-equity-playbook-how-city -leaders-can-bridge-the-digital-divide?id=3.

48. United Way NCA, "Analyzing Digital Equity in America," Feb. 6, 2023, https://unitedwaynca.org/blog/analyzing-digital-equity-in-america/.

49. Green & Healthy Homes Initiative, "About Us," https://www.greenand healthyhomes.org/about-us/.

50. Ruth Ann Norton and Brendan Brown, "Improving Health, Economic, and Social Outcomes Through Integrated Housing Intervention," *Environmental Justice* 7, no. 6 (2014): 151–57, doi: 10.1089/env.2014.0033.

51. Elizabeth Fussell, Narayan Sastry, and Mark Vanlandingham, "Race, Socioeconomic Status, and Return Migration to New Orleans After Hurricane Katrina," *Population and Environment* 31 (2010): 20–42, doi: 10.1007/s11111-009-0092-2.

52. Federal Emergency Management, "Achieving Equitable Recovery: A Post-Disaster Guide for Local Officials and Leaders," Nov. 2023, https://www.fema.gov /sites/default/files/documents/fema_equitable-recovery-post-disaster-guide-local -officials-leaders.pdf; Ritwik Gupta, Shankar Sastry, Janet Napolitano, and Berkeley Center for Science and Technology Policy, "Trustworthy Disaster Response Technology," Center for Security in Politics, University of California Berkeley, https://csp.berkeley.edu/2023/10/17/trustworthy-disaster-response-technology -policy-and-society/.

53. Abdul-Akeem Sadiq, Jenna Tyler, and Douglas S. Noonan, "A Review of Community Flood Risk Management Studies in the United States," *International Journal of Disaster Risk Reduction* 41 (2019): 101327, doi: 10.1016/j.ijdrr.2019 .101327.

CHAPTER FOUR: LIVING ON THE MARGINS

1. Dorothy Oliver, interview by Monica Wang, virtual, Boston, MA, May 5, 2022.

2. James C. Davis et al., *Rural America at a Glance: 2023 Edition*, Economic Research Service, US Department of Agriculture, https://www.ers.usda.gov/web docs/publications/107838/eib-261.pdf/, doi.org/10.32747/2023.8134362.ers.

3. US Federal Reserve, *Changes in U.S. Family Finances from 2019 to 2022: Evidence from the Survey of Consumer Finances*, Oct. 2023, https://www.federalreserve .gov/publications/files/scf23.pdf.

4. Kenneth Johnson and Daniel Lichter, "Growing Racial Diversity in Rural America: Results from the 2020 Census," Carsey School of Public Policy, University of New Hampshire, May 25, 2022, https://carsey.unh.edu/publication/growing -racial-diversity-rural-america-results-2020-census.

5. Economic Research Service, US Department of Agriculture, "Rural Poverty & Well-Being: Demographics," Nov. 15, 2023, https://www.ers.usda.gov/topics /rural-economy-population/rural-poverty-well-being/#demographics.

6. Rural Health Information Hub, "Healthcare Access in Rural Communities," last updated Dec. 19, 2024, https://www.ruralhealthinfo.org/topics/healthcare -access.

7. Marvellous Akinlotan et al., "Rural-Urban Variations in Travel Burdens for Care: Findings from the 2017 National Household Travel Survey," Southwest Rural Health Research Center, July 2021, https://srhrc.tamu.edu/publications /rural-urban-variations-in-travel-burdens-for-care-policy-brief07.2021.pdf.

8. "Rural Health," *Health Affairs* 38, no. 12 (2019): 1964–65, doi: 10.1377 /hlthaff.2019.01365.

9. Economic Research Service, US Department of Agriculture, "Availability of Healthcare Providers in Rural Areas Lags That of Urban Areas," Apr. 3, 2023, https://www.ers.usda.gov/data-products/chart-gallery/gallery/chart-detail/?chart Id=106208.

10. Cecil G. Sheps Center for Health Services Research, "171 Rural Hospital Closures: January 2005–Present (129 Since 2010)," University of North Carolina, http://www.shepscenter.unc.edu/programs-projects/rural-health/rural-hospital -closures/.

11. Austin B. Frakt, "The Rural Hospital Problem," *JAMA* 321, no. 23 (2019): 2271–72.

12. Mary Kakatos, "Rural Americans Are at Higher Risk of Early Death Than Urbanites: CDC," ABC News, Apr. 30, 2024, https://abcnews.go.com/Health /rural-americans-higher-risk-early-death-urbanites-cdc/story?id=109742216.

13. Rural Health Information Hub, "Healthcare Access in Rural Communities," last updated Dec. 19, 2024, https://www.ruralhealthinfo.org/topics/healthcare -access.

14. Samina T. Syed, Ben S. Gerber, and Lisa K. Sharp, "Traveling Towards Disease: Transportation Barriers to Health Care Access," *Journal of Community Health* 38, no. 5 (2013): 976–93, doi: 10.1007/s10900-013-9681-1.

15. Munira Z. Gunja, "Rural Americans Struggle with Medical Bills and Health Care Affordability," *To the Point* (blog), Commonwealth Fund, July 24, 2023, https://doi.org/10.26099/pq3a-k123.

16. David W. Schopfer, "Rural Health Disparities in Chronic Heart Disease," *Preventive Medicine* 152, pt. 2 (2021): 106782, doi: 10.1016/j.ypmed.2021.106782.

17. National Institute for Health Care Management Foundation, "Rural Health: Addressing Barriers to Care," Oct. 25, 2023, https://nihcm.org/publication /rural-health-addressing-barriers-to-care.

18. Sophia Campbell, Jimena Ruiz Castro, and David Wessel, "The Benefits and Costs of Broadband Expansion," Brookings Institute, Aug. 18, 2021, https:// www.brookings.edu/articles/the-benefits-and-costs-of-broadband-expansion/.

19. Federal Communications Commission, *2020 Broadband Deployment Report*, June 8, 2020, https://www.fcc.gov/reports-research/reports/broadband-progress -reports/2020-broadband-deployment-report.

20. Emily A. Vogels, "Some Digital Divides Persist Between Rural, Urban, and Suburban America," Pew Research Center, Aug. 19, 2021, https://www.pewresearch .org/short-reads/2021/08/19/some-digital-divides-persist-between-rural-urban -and-suburban-america/.

21. Zachary Levinson, Jamie Godwin, and Scott Hulver, "Rural Hospitals Face Renewed Financial Challenges, Especially in States That Have Not Expanded Medicaid," Kaiser Family Foundation, Feb. 23, 2023, https://www.kff.org/health -costs/issue-brief/rural-hospitals-face-renewed-financial-challenges-especially -in-states-that-have-not-expanded-medicaid/.

22. Eunji Kim, Michael E. Shepherd, and Joshua D. Clinton, "The Effect of Big-City News on Rural America During the COVID-19 Pandemic," *Proceedings of the National Academy of Sciences U.S.A.* 117, no. 36 (2020): 22009–22014, doi: 10.1073/pnas .2009384117; Elizabeth Griecco, "For Many Rural Residents in U.S., Local News Media Mostly Don't Cover the Area Where They Live," Pew Research Center, Apr. 12, 2019, https://www.pewresearch.org/short-reads/2019/04/12/for-many-rural -residents-in-u-s-local-news-media-mostly-dont-cover-the-area-where-they-live/.

23. David S. Jones, "The Persistence of American Indian Health Disparities," *American Journal of Public Health* 96, no. 12 (2006): 2122–34, doi: 10.2105/AJPH .2004.054262; Karina L. Walters et al., "Dis-placement and Dis-ease: Land, Place, and Health Among American Indians and Alaska Natives," in *Communities, Neighborhoods, and Health*, ed. L. Burton, S. Matthews, M. Leung, S. Kemp, and D. Takeuchi (New York: Springer, 2011).

24. Margery A. Turner and Solomon Greene, *Causes and Consequences of Separate and Unequal Neighborhoods*, Urban Institute, https://www.urban.org/racial -equity-analytics-lab/structural-racism-explainer-collection/causes-and -consequences-separate-and-unequal-neighborhoods, accessed Feb. 19, 2025.

25. Cara V. James et al., "Racial/Ethnic Health Disparities Among Rural Adults—United States, 2012–2015," *MMWR Surveillance Summaries* 66, no. SS-23 (2017): 1–9, doi: 10.15585/mmwr.ss6623a1.

26. H. Joanna Jiang et al., "Mortality for Time-Sensitive Conditions at Urban vs. Rural Hospitals During the COVID-19 Pandemic," *JAMA Network Open* 7, no. 3 (2024): e241838, doi:10.1001/jamanetworkopen.2024.1838; Alfred Anzalone et al. and the National Consortium, "Higher Hospitalization and Mortality Rates Among SARS-CoV-2-Infected Persons in Rural America," *Journal of Rural Health* 39, no. 1 (2023): 39–54, doi: 10.1111/jrh.12689.

27. Shawnda Schroeder, "Rural Communities: Age, Income, and Health Status," Rural Health Research RECAP, Rural Health Research Gateway, Nov. 2018, https://www.ruralhealthresearch.org/assets/2200-8536/rural-communities-age -income-health-status-recap.pdf.

28. J. Tom Mueller et al., "Impacts of the COVID-19 Pandemic on Rural America," *Proceedings of the National Academy of Sciences U.S.A.* 118, no. 1 (2021): 2019378118, doi: 10.1073/pnas.2019378118.

29. Diego F. Cuadros et al., "Dynamics of the COVID-19 Epidemic in Urban and Rural Areas in the United States," *Annals of Epidemiology* 59 (July 2021): 16–20, doi: 10.1016/j.annepidem.2021.04.007.

30. National Telecommunications and Information Administration, "Digital Equity Act Programs," https://broadbandusa.ntia.doc.gov/funding-programs /digital-equity-act-programs.

31. US Congress, *S.1162—Accurate Map for Broadband Investment Act of 2023*, introduced May 30, 2023, https://www.congress.gov/bill/118th-congress/senate -bill/1162.

32. State of California, "About Broadband for All," https://broadbandforall.cdt
.ca.gov/about/.

33. Pew Charitable Trusts, "What Policymakers Can Learn from the 'Minnesota Model' of Broadband Expansion," Mar. 2, 2021, https://www.pewtrusts.org
/en/research-and-analysis/articles/2021/03/02/what-policymakers-can-learn-from
-the-minnesota-model-of-broadband-expansion.

34. Broadband USA, "Maine Becomes First State to Have Digital Equity
Plan Accepted," National Telecommunications and Information Administration,
https://broadbandusa.ntia.doc.gov/news/latest-news/maine-becomes-first-state
-have-digital-equity-plan-accepted.

35. Annie E. Larson et al., "Before and During Pandemic Telemedicine Use:
An Analysis of Rural and Urban Safety-Net Clinics," *American Journal of Preventive Medicine* 63, no. 6 (2022): 1031–36, doi: 10.1016/j.amepre.2022.06.012.

36. Consolidated Appropriations Act of 2021, Pub. L. No. 116–260, 134 Stat.
1182 (2020), available at https://www.govinfo.gov/content/pkg/PLAW-116publ260
/pdf/PLAW-116publ260.pdf; Sara L. Schaefer, Cody L. Mullens, and Andrew M.
Ibrahim, "The Emergence of Rural Emergency Hospitals: Safely Implementing
New Models of Care," *JAMA* 329, no. 13 (2023): 1059–60, doi: 10.1001/jama
.2023.1956.

37. Yasmin Khan et al., "Public Health Emergency Preparedness: A Framework to Promote Resilience," *BMC Public Health* 18 (2018): 1344, doi: 10.1186
/s12889-018-6250-7.

38. Rural Health Information Hub, "Social Determinants of Health for
Rural People," https://www.ruralhealthinfo.org/topics/social-determinants-of
-health.

CHAPTER FIVE: THE STRENGTH OF WEAK TIES

1. Latoya Hill and Samantha Artiga, *COVID-19 Cases and Deaths by Race/
Ethnicity: Current Data and Changes Over Time*, Kaiser Family Foundation, Aug. 2,
2022, https://www.kff.org/racial-equity-and-health-policy/issue-brief/covid-19
-cases-and-deaths-by-race-ethnicity-current-data-and-changes-over-time/;
COVID Tracking Project, COVID Racial Data Tracker, https://covidtracking
.com/race.

2. Lisa F. Berkman and Aditi Krishna, "Social Network Epidemiology," in
Social Epidemiology, 2nd ed., ed. Lisa F. Berkman, Ichiro Kawachi, and M. Maria
Glymour (New York: Oxford Academic, 2015).

3. Lisa F. Berkman and S. Leonard Syme, "Social Networks, Host Resistance,
and Mortality: A Nine-Year Follow-Up Study of Alameda County Residents,"
American Journal of Epidemiology 109, no. 2 (Feb. 1979): 186–204, doi: 10.1093
/oxfordjournals.aje.a112674.

4. Ichiro Kawachi et al., "A Prospective Study of Social Networks in Relation
to Total Mortality and Cardiovascular Disease in Men in the USA," *Journal of
Epidemiology and Community Health* 50, no. 3 (June 1996): 245–51, doi: 10.1136
/jech.50.3.245.

5. Priya J. Wickramaratne et al., "Social Connectedness as a Determinant
of Mental Health: A Scoping Review," *PLOS ONE* 17, no. 10 (Oct. 13, 2022):
e0275004, doi: 10.1371/journal.pone.0275004.

6. Claire Y. Yang et al., "Social Relationships and Physiological Determinants of Longevity Across the Human Life Span," *Proceedings of the National Academy of Sciences* 113, no. 3 (2016): 578–83, doi: 10.1073/pnas.1511085112.

7. Lisa F. Berkman and Lester Breslow, *Health and Ways of Living: The Alameda County Study* (New York: Oxford University Press, 1983); Debra Umberson and Jennifer K. Montez, "Social Relationships and Health: A Flashpoint for Health Policy," *Journal of Health and Social Behavior* 51, Suppl. (2010): S54–S66, doi: 10.1177/0022146510383501.

8. Andrew S. Proctor, Abigail Barth, and Julianne Holt-Lunstad, "A Healthy Lifestyle Is a Social Lifestyle: The Vital Link Between Social Connection and Health Outcomes," *Lifestyle Medicine* 4 (2023): e91.b, doi: 10.1002/lim2.91; Julianne Holt-Lunstad, "Why Social Relationships Are Important for Physical Health: A Systems Approach to Understanding and Modifying Risk and Protection," *Annual Review of Psychology* 69 (2018): 437–58, doi: 10.1146/annurev-psych-122216-011902; Julianne Holt-Lunstad, Timothy B. Smith, and J. Bradley Layton, "Social Relationships and Mortality Risk: A Meta-Analytic Review," *PLOS Medicine* 7, no. 7 (July 27, 2010): e1000316, doi: 10.1371/journal.pmed.1000316.

9. Mary E. Procidano and Kenneth Heller, "Measures of Perceived Social Support from Friends and from Family: Three Validation Studies," *American Journal of Community Psychology* 11, no. 1 (1983): 1–24, doi: 10.1007/BF00898416.

10. Maija Reblin and Bert N. Uchino, "Social and Emotional Support and Its Implication for Health," *Current Opinion in Psychiatry* 21, no. 2 (Mar. 2008): 201–5, doi: 10.1097/YCO.0b013e3282f3ad89; Bert N. Uchino, "Social Support and Health: A Review of Physiological Processes Potentially Underlying Links to Disease Outcomes," *Journal of Behavioral Medicine* 29, no. 4 (Aug. 2006): 377–87, doi: 10.1007/s10865-006-9056-5.

11. Lisa F. Berkman, Linda Leo-Summers, and Ralph I. Horwitz, "Emotional Support and Survival After Myocardial Infarction: A Prospective, Population-Based Study of the Elderly," *Annals of Internal Medicine* 117, no. 12 (Dec. 15, 1992): 1003–9, doi: 10.7326/0003-4819-117-12-1003.

12. Robert G. Kent de Grey et al., "Social Support," *Oxford Bibliographies in Psychology*, 2018, doi: 10.1093/OBO/9780199828340-0204.

13. Jorunn Drageset, "Social Support," in *Health Promotion in Health Care—Vital Theories and Research*, ed. G. Haugan and M. Eriksson (Cham: Springer, 2021), https://www.ncbi.nlm.nih.gov/books/NBK585650/, doi:10.1007/978-3-030-63135-2_11.

14. Monica L. Wang, Olivia J. Britton, and Jennifer Beard, "The Call for Science Communication and Public Scholarship," *Translational Behavioral Medicine* 13, no. 3 (Apr. 3, 2023): 156–59, doi:10.1093/tbm/ibac096; Carly M. Goldstein et al., "Science Communication in the Age of Misinformation," *Annals of Behavioral Medicine* 54, no. 12 (Dec. 1, 2020): 985–90, doi:10.1093/abm/kaaa088.

15. Tiansheng Xia et al., "The Relationship Between Career Social Support and Employability of College Students: A Moderated Mediation Model," *Frontiers in Psychology* 11 (Jan. 28, 2020): 28, doi: 10.3389/fpsyg.2020.00028.

16. Beth E. Schultz, Cynthia F. Corbett, and Ronda G. Hughes, "Instrumental Support: A Conceptual Analysis," *Nursing Forum* 57, no. 4 (July 2022): 665–70, doi:10.1111/nuf.12704; epub Feb. 8, 2022, doi: 10.1111/nuf.12704.

17. Monica L. Wang, Lori Pbert, and Stephenie C. Lemon, "Influence of Family, Friend, and Coworker Social Support and Social Undermining on Weight Gain Prevention Among Adults," *Obesity* 22, no. 9 (Sept. 2014): 1973–80.

18. Ichiro Kawachi and Lisa F. Berkman, "Social Ties and Mental Health," *Journal of Urban Health* 78, no. 3 (Sept. 2001): 458–67, doi: 10.1093/jurban/78.3.458.

19. Suzanne Higgs, "Social Norms and Their Influence on Eating Behaviors," *Appetite* 86C (2014): 38–44, doi: 10.1016/j.appet.2014.10.021; Kylie Ball et al., "Is Healthy Behavior Contagious: Associations of Social Norms with Physical Activity and Healthy Eating," *International Journal of Behavioral Nutrition and Physical Activity* 7 (2010): 86, doi: 10.1186/1479-5868-7-86.

20. Susan T. Ennett et al., "The Peer Context of Adolescent Substance Use: Findings from Social Network Analysis," *Journal of Research on Adolescence* 16, no. 2 (2006): 159–86, doi: 10.1111/j.1532-7795.2006.00127.x; Carl A. Latkin et al., "Norms, Social Networks, and HIV-Related Risk Behaviors Among Urban Disadvantaged Drug Users," *Social Science & Medicine* 56, no. 3 (Feb. 2003): 465–76, doi: 10.1016/S0277-9536(02)00047-3.

21. Nicholas A. Christakis and James H. Fowler, "The Spread of Obesity in a Large Social Network Over 32 Years," *New England Journal of Medicine* 357 (2007): 370–79, doi: 10.1056/NEJMsa066082.

22. Nicholas A. Christakis and James H. Fowler, "The Collective Dynamics of Smoking in a Large Social Network," *New England Journal of Medicine* 358, no. 21 (May 22, 2008): 2249–58, doi: 10.1056/NEJMsa0706154.

23. Sinan Aral and Christos Nicolaides, "Exercise Contagion in a Global Social Network," *Nature Communications* 8 (2017): 14753, doi: 10.1038/ncomms14753.

24. J. Niels Rosenquist et al., "The Spread of Alcohol Consumption Behavior in a Large Social Network," *Annals of Internal Medicine* 152, no. 7 (Apr. 6, 2010): 426–33, W141, doi: 10.7326/0003-4819-152-7-201004060-00007.

25. Pinelopi Konstantinou et al., "Transmission of Vaccination Attitudes and Uptake Based on Social Contagion Theory: A Scoping Review," *Vaccines* 9, no. 6 (June 5, 2021): 607, doi: 10.3390/vaccines9060607.

26. National Research Council (US), Committee on Aging Frontiers in Social Psychology, Personality, and Adult Developmental Psychology; and L. L. Carstensen and C. R. Hartel, eds., *When I'm 64* (Washington, DC: National Academies Press, 2006), https://www.ncbi.nlm.nih.gov/books/NBK83766/.

27. Mengyun Luo et al., "Social Engagement Pattern, Health Behaviors, and Subjective Well-Being of Older Adults: An International Perspective Using WHO-SAGE Survey Data," *BMC Public Health* 20 (2020): 99, doi: 10.1186/s12889-019-7841-7; Peter A. Bath and Dorly Deeg, "Social Engagement and Health Outcomes Among Older People: Introduction to a Special Section," *European Journal of Ageing* 2, no. 1 (Mar. 2005): 24–30, doi: 10.1007/s10433-005-0019-4.

28. Nexhmedin Morina et al., "Potential Impact of Physical Distancing on Physical and Mental Health: A Rapid Narrative Umbrella Review of Meta-Analyses on the Link Between Social Connection and Health," *BMJ Open* 11, no. 3 (2021): e042335, doi: 10.1136/bmjopen-2020-042335; Matthew T. Tull

et al., "Psychological Outcomes Associated with Stay-at-Home Orders and the Perceived Impact of COVID-19 on Daily Life," *Psychiatry Research* 289 (2020): 113098, doi: 10.1016/j.psychres.2020.113098.

29. Ming-Te Wang et al., "Social Distancing and Adolescent Psychological Well-Being: The Role of Practical Knowledge and Exercise," *Academic Pediatrics* 22, no. 3 (Apr. 2022): 402–12, doi: 10.1016/j.acap.2021.10.008; Benjamin Oosterhoff et al., "Adolescents' Motivations to Engage in Social Distancing During the COVID-19 Pandemic: Associations with Mental and Social Health," *Journal of Adolescent Health* (2020): 1–7, doi: 10.1016/j.jadohealth.2020.05.004.

30. Jörg M. Fegert et al., "Challenges and Burden of the Coronavirus 2019 (COVID-19) Pandemic for Child and Adolescent Mental Health: A Narrative Review to Highlight Clinical and Research Needs in the Acute Phase and the Long Return to Normality," *Child and Adolescent Psychiatry and Mental Health* 14 (2020): 20, doi: 10.1186/s13034-020-00329-3.

31. Mark S. Granovetter, "The Strength of Weak Ties," *American Journal of Sociology* 78 (1973): 1360–80, http://www.jstor.org/stable/2776392.

32. Maarit Kauppi et al., "Characteristics of Social Networks and Mortality Risk: Evidence from 2 Prospective Cohort Studies," *American Journal of Epidemiology* 187, no. 4 (Apr. 1, 2018): 746–53, doi: 10.1093/aje/kwx301.

33. Ichiro Kawachi and Lisa F. Berkman, "Social Capital, Social Cohesion, and Health," in *Social Epidemiology*, 2nd ed., ed. Lisa F. Berkman, Ichiro Kawachi, and Maria M. Glymour (New York: Oxford Academic, 2014), doi: 10.1093/med /9780195377903.003.0008.

34. Ichiro Kawachi et al., "Social Capital, Income Inequality, and Mortality," *American Journal of Public Health* 87, no. 9 (Sept. 1997): 1491–98, doi:10.2105/ajph .87.9.1491.

35. Yang Han and Roger Yat-Nork Chung, "The Role of Neighborhood Social Capital on Health and Health Inequality in Rural and Urban China," *Preventive Medicine* 156 (Mar. 2022): 106989, doi: 10.1016/j.ypmed.2022.106989.

36. Robert D. Putnam, "Social Capital and Public Affairs," *Bulletin of the American Academy of Arts and Sciences* 47, no. 8 (1994): 5–19, doi: 10.2307/3824796.

37. Robert D. Putnam, *Democracies in Flux: The Evolution of Social Capital in Contemporary Society* (New York: Oxford Academic, 2002), doi: 10.1093/0195150899 .001.0001.

38. Eric Klinenberg, *Heat Wave: A Social Autopsy of Disaster in Chicago*, 2nd ed. (Chicago: University of Chicago Press, 2015).

39. Simon Szreter and Michael Woolcock, "Health by Association? Social Capital, Social Theory, and the Political Economy of Public Health," *International Journal of Epidemiology* 33, no. 4 (2004): 650–67, doi: 10.1093/ije/dyh013.

40. Elizabeth Fussell, Narayan Sastry, and Mark Vanlandingham, "Race, Socioeconomic Status, and Return Migration to New Orleans after Hurricane Katrina," *Population and Environment* 31, no. 1–3 (Jan. 2010): 20–42, doi:10.1007 /s11111-009-0092-2.

41. Manning Marable and Kristen Clarke-Avery, *Seeking Higher Ground: The Hurricane Katrina Crisis, Race, and Public Policy Reader* (New York: Palgrave Macmillan, 2008).

42. Robert L. Hawkins and Katherine Maurer, "Bonding, Bridging, and Linking: How Social Capital Operated in New Orleans Following Hurricane Katrina," *British Journal of Social Work* 40, no. 6 (2010): 1777–93, doi: 10.1093/bjsw/bcp087.

43. Pat Crawford et al., "Social Capital Development in Participatory Community Planning and Design," *Town Planning Review* 79 (2008): 533–54, doi:10.3828/tpr.79.5.5; E. Villalonga-Olives, T. R. Wind, and I. Kawachi, "Social Capital Interventions in Public Health: A Systematic Review," *Social Science & Medicine* 212 (Sept. 2018): 203–18, doi: 10.1016/j.socscimed.2018.07.022.

44. Caitlin Eicher and Ichiro Kawachi, "Social Capital and Community Design," in *Making Healthy Places: Designing and Building for Health, Well-being, and Sustainability*, ed. Andrew L. Dannenberg, Howard Frumkin, and Richard J. Jackson (Washington, DC: Island Press, 2011), 8.

45. American Planning Association, Washington Chapter, Social Capital Group, *Building Social Capital Through Urban Design and Planning Activities*, https://www.washington-apa.org/assets/docs/2015/Ten_Big_Ideas/21_%20updated%20use%20this%20version%20big%20ideas%20social%20capital%20report.pdf.

46. Lisa Dang et al., "Explaining Civic Engagement: The Role of Neighborhood Ties, Place Attachment, and Civic Responsibility," *Journal of Community Psychology* 50, no. 3 (2022): 1736–55, doi: 10.1002/jcop.22751.

47. Isabel V. Sawhill, "Social Capital: Why We Need It and How We Can Create More of It," Brookings Institute, July 2020, https://www.brookings.edu/wp-content/uploads/2020/07/Sawhill_Social-Capital_Final_07.16.2020.pdf.

48. Marco Ambrosio, Chris Bullivant, Patrick Brown, Jane Oates, and Peyton Roth, and Social Capital Campaign, *Social Capital Works*, Dec. 2022, https://static1.squarespace.com/static/60abb375ca5a79523fb94711/t/639b64ae8ce4a71a8782c434/1671128240234/SCC-SocialCapitalWorks.pdf.

49. K. Hazel Kwon, "The Analysis of Social Capital in Digital Environments: A Social Investment Approach," in *The Oxford Handbook of Networked Communication*, ed. Brooke Foucault Welles and Sandra González-Bailón, Oxford Handbooks (2020; online ed., Oxford Academic, Apr. 2018), doi: 10.1093/oxfordhb/9780190460518.013.14.

50. Krystian Siebert, "Celeste Barber's Story Shows Us the Power of Celebrity Fundraising … and the Importance of Reading the Fine Print," *The Conversation*, May 26, 2020, https://theconversation.com/celeste-barbers-story-shows-us-the-power-of-celebrity-fundraising-and-the-importance-of-reading-the-fine-print-139379.

51. ALS Association, "Raising Ice Buckets to Raise ALS Awareness," May 1, 2024, https://www.als.org/blog/raising-ice-buckets-raise-als-awareness.

CHAPTER SIX: WHAT'S IN A NAME?

1. World Health Organization, "Pneumonia of Unknown Cause—China," *Disease Outbreak News*, Jan. 5, 2020, https://www.who.int/emergencies/disease-outbreak-news/item/2020-DON229.

2. Sui-Lee Wee and Donald G. McNeil Jr., "China Confirms Pneumonia Outbreak," *New York Times*, Jan. 8, 2020, https://www.nytimes.com/2020/01/08/health/china-pneumonia-outbreak-virus.html.

3. Centers for Disease Control and Prevention, "COVID-19 Timeline," CDC Museum, 2020, https://www.cdc.gov/museum/timeline/covid19.html.

4. Björn P. Zietz and Hartmut Dunkelberg, "The History of the Plague and the Research on the Causative Agent Yersinia Pestis," *International Journal of Hygiene and Environmental Health* 207, no. 2 (2004): 165–78, doi: 10.1078/1438 -4639-00259; Frank R. DeLeo and B. Joseph Hinnebusch, "A Plague upon the Phagocytes," *Nature Medicine* 11, no. 9 (2005): 927–28, doi: 10.1038/nm0905-927.

5. Samuel K. K. Cohn Jr., "The Black Death and the Burning of Jews," *Past & Present* 196, no. 1 (2007): 3–36, doi: 10.1093/pastj/gtm005.

6. Anna Foa, *The Jews of Europe After the Black Death* (Berkeley: University of California Press, 2000).

7. Michael Omer-Man, "This Week in History: The Jews of Basel Are Burnt," *Jerusalem Post*, Apr. 2011.

8. Albert Winkler, "The Medieval Holocaust: The Approach of the Plague and the Destruction of Jews in Germany, 1348–1349," *Brigham Young University Scholars Archive Faculty Publications* (2005): 1816, https://scholarsarchive.byu.edu /facpub/1816.

9. D. W. Williams, "The Germ-Theory," *BMJ* 1, no. 536 (1871): 368, doi: 10.1136/bmj.1.536.368.

10. P. Smit and J. Heniger, "Antoni Van Leeuwenhoek (1632–1723) and the Discovery of Bacteria," *Antonie Van Leeuwenhoek* 41, no. 1 (1975): 217–28, doi: 10.3390/microorganisms11081994.

11. Hervé Lecoq, "Découverte du premier virus, le virus de la mosaïque du tabac: 1892 ou 1898?" *Comptes Rendus de l'Académie des Sciences–Series III–Sciences de la Vie* 324, no. 10 (2001): 929–33, doi: 10.1016/s0764-4469(01)01368-3.

12. Bernard N. Fields, David M. Knipe, and Peter M. Howley, *Fields Virology*, 5th ed. (Philadelphia: Wolters Kluwer Health/Lippincott Williams & Wilkins, 2007).

13. Matthew I. Hutchings, Andrew W. Truman, and Barrie Wilkinson, "Antibiotics: Past, Present and Future," *Current Opinion in Microbiology* 51 (2019): 72–80, doi: 10.1016/j.mib.2019.10.008; Alexandra Minna Stern and Howard Markel, "The History of Vaccines and Immunization: Familiar Patterns, New Challenges," *Health Affairs* 24, no. 3 (2005): 611–21, doi: 10.1377/hlthaff.24.3.611.

14. Jeffery K. Taubenberger and David M. Morens, "The 1918 Influenza Pandemic and Its Legacy," *Cold Spring Harbor Perspectives in Medicine* 10, no. 10 (2020): a038695, doi: 10.1101/cshperspect.a038695.

15. Antoni Trilla, Guillem Trilla, and Carolyn Daer, "The 1918 'Spanish Flu' in Spain," *Clinical Infectious Diseases* 47, no. 5 (2008): 668–73, doi: 10.1086/590567.

16. Trevor Hoppe, "'Spanish Flu': When Infectious Disease Names Blur Origins and Stigmatize Those Infected," *American Journal of Public Health* 108, no. 11 (2018): 1462–64, doi: 10.2105/AJPH.2018.304645.

17. Tilli Tansey, "Influenza: A Viral World War," *Nature* 546, no. 7657 (2017): 207–8, doi: 10.1038/546207a.

18. Iain Marlow, "Trump's Retweet of 'China Virus' Term Sparks Backlash, Fuels Tensions with Beijing," *Time*, Mar. 11, 2020.

19. Stanford M. Lyman, "The 'Yellow Peril' Mystique: Origins and Vicissitudes of a Racist Discourse," *International Journal of Politics, Culture, and Society* 13, no. 4 (2000): 683–747, doi: 10.1023/A:1022931309651.

20. Michael Lee, "When Chinese Americans Were Scapegoated for Bubonic Plague," History.com, Oct. 11, 2022, https://www.history.com/news/bubonic -plague-honolulu-fire-san-francisco.

21. Donna K. Nagata, Jacqueline H. J. Kim, and Kaidi Wu, "The Japanese American Wartime Incarceration: Examining the Scope of Racial Trauma," *American Psychologist* 74, no. 1 (2019): 36–48, doi: 10.1037/amp0000303.

22. "Fishing Town in Texas Tells the Klan to Stay Away," *New York Times*, Nov. 22, 1979.

23. Frank H. Wu, "Embracing Mistaken Identity: How the Vincent Chin Case Unified Asian Americans," *Asian American Policy Review* 19 (2010): 17.

24. J. S. Peiris et al. and the SARS Study Group, "Coronavirus as a Possible Cause of Severe Acute Respiratory Syndrome," *The Lancet* 361, no. 9366 (2003): 1319–25, doi: 10.1016/s0140-6736(03)13077-2; World Health Organization, "Severe Acute Respiratory Syndrome (SARS)," https://www.who.int/health-topics /severe-acute-respiratory-syndrome.

25. Laura Eichelberger, "SARS and New York's Chinatown: The Politics of Risk and Blame during an Epidemic of Fear," *Social Science & Medicine* 65, no. 6 (2007): 1284–95, doi: 10.1016/j.socscimed.2007.04.022.

26. Jennifer Lee and Dean E. Murphy, "The SARS Epidemic: Asian-Americans; In U.S., Fear Is Spreading Faster Than SARS," *New York Times*, Apr. 17, 2003, https://www.nytimes.com/2003/04/17/world/the-sars-epidemic -asian-americans-in-us-fear-is-spreading-faster-than-sars.html.

27. Centers for Disease Control and Prevention, "Revised U.S. Surveillance Case Definition for Severe Acute Respiratory Syndrome (SARS) and Update on SARS Cases—United States and Worldwide, December 2003," *Morbidity and Mortality Weekly Report* 52, no. 49 (2003): 1202–6.

28. Adrian J. Gibbs, John S. Armstrong, and Jean C. Downie, "From Where Did the 2009 'Swine-Origin' Influenza A Virus (H1N1) Emerge?" *Virology Journal* 6, no. 1 (2009), doi: 10.1186/1743-422X-6-207.

29. Media Matters Staff, "Boortz Suggests Renaming the 'Swine Flu,' the 'Fajita Flu,'" Media Matters for America, Apr. 29, 2009.

30. Media Matters Staff, "Discussing 'Outbreak of Swine Flu, or H1N1 Virus, or the Mexican Flu, or Whatever,' Dobbs Calls Those Using H1N1 Terminology 'Idiots,'" Media Matters for America, Apr. 29, 2009.

31. Michael McCauley, Sara Minsky, and Kasisomayajula Viswanath, "The H1N1 Pandemic: Media Frames, Stigmatization and Coping," *BMC Public Health* 13, no. 1 (2013), doi: 10.1186/1471-2458-13-1116.

32. Monica Schoch-Spana et al., "Stigma, Health Disparities, and the 2009 H1N1 Influenza Pandemic: How to Protect Latino Farmworkers in Future Health Emergencies," *Biosecurity and Bioterrorism: Biodefense Strategy, Practice, and Science* 8, no. 3 (2010): 243–54, doi: 10.1089/bsp.2010.0021.

33. Center for the Study of Hate and Extremism, "Anti-Asian Hate Fact Sheet," California State University, San Bernardino, 2020, https://www.csusb.edu/sites default/files/FACT%20SHEET-%20Anti-Asian%20Hate%202020%203.2.21.pdf.

34. Neil G. Ruiz, Caroline Im, and Ziyao Tian, "Asian Americans and the Model Minority Stereotype," Pew Research Center, Nov. 30, 2023, https://www .pewresearch.org/2023/11/30/asian-americans-and-the-model-minority-stereotype/.

35. Abby Budiman, "Hmong in the U.S. Fact Sheet," Pew Research Center, Apr. 29, 2021, https://www.pewresearch.org/fact-sheet/asian-americans-hmong -in-the-u-s/.

36. Abby Budiman and Neil G. Ruiz, "Key Facts about Asian Americans," Pew Research Center, Apr. 29, 2021, https://www.pewresearch.org/short-reads/2021 /04/29/key-facts-about-asian-americans/.

37. Tiffany Wang et al., "Working w Burmese Patients: Understanding Historical and Cultural Contexts to Improve Health Care Access and Health Status," *MedEdPORTAL* 18 (2022): 11260, doi: 10.15766/mep_2374-8265.11260.

38. Andy Menke et al., "Prevalence of and Trends in Diabetes Among Adults in the United States, 1988–2012," *JAMA* 314, no. 10 (2015): 1021–29, doi:10.1001/jama.2015.10029; Michael Fang et al., "Undiagnosed Diabetes in U.S. Adults: Prevalence and Trends," *Diabetes Care* 45, no. 9 (2022): 1994–2002, doi: 10.2337/dc22-0242.

39. Richard J. Lee et al., "Disparities in Cancer Care and the Asian American Population," *Oncologist* 26, no. 6 (2021): 453–60, doi: 10.1002/onco.13748.

40. Hongbin Jin et al., "Cancer Incidence Among Asian American Populations in the United States, 2009-2011," *International Journal of Cancer* 138, no. 9 (2016): 2136–45, doi: 10.1002/ijc.29958.

41. Mindy C. DeRouen et al., "Incidence of Lung Cancer Among Never-Smoking Asian American, Native Hawaiian, and Pacific Islander Females," *Journal of the National Cancer Institute* 114, no. 1 (2022): 78–86, doi: 10.1093/jnci/djab143.

42. Moon S. Chen et al., "Charting a Path Towards Asian American Cancer Health Equity: A Way Forward," *JNCI: Journal of the National Cancer Institute* 114, no. 6 (2022): 792–99, doi: 10.1093/jnci/djaco55; Victoria Colliver, "New UCSF Study to Find Out What Drives Cancer in Asian Americans," University of California, San Francisco, May 21, 2024, https://www.ucsf.edu/news/2024/05/427586 /new-ucsf-study-find-out-what-drives-cancer-asian-americans.

43. Hyeouk Chris Hahm et al., "Perceived COVID-19-Related Anti-Asian Discrimination Predicts Post-Traumatic Stress Disorder Symptoms Among Asian and Asian American Young Adults," *Psychiatry Research* 303 (2021): 114084, doi: 10.1016/j.psychres.2021.114084; Jusung Lee and Jeffrey T. Howard, "Increased Self-Reported Mental Health Problems Among Asian Americans During the COVID-19 Pandemic in the United States: Evidence from a Nationally Representative Database," *Journal of Racial and Ethnic Health Disparities* 10, no. 5 (2023): 2344–53, doi: 10.1007/s40615-022-01414-3.

44. Astraea Augsberger et al., "Factors Influencing the Underutilization of Mental Health Services Among Asian American Women with a History of Depression and Suicide," *BMC Health Services Research* 15, no. 1 (2015): 542; Stanley Sue et al., "Asian American Mental Health: A Call to Action," *American Psychologist* 67, no. 7 (2012): 532–44, doi: 10.1037/a0028900.

45. Ellen R. Huang and Gordon C. Nagayama Hall, "The Invisibility of Asian Americans in the United States: Impact on Mental and Physical Health," in *Prejudice, Stigma, Privilege, and Oppression*, ed. L. Benuto, M. Duckworth, A. Masuda, and W. O'Donohue (Cham: Springer, 2020), doi: 10.1007/978-3-030 -35517-3_6.

46. Lindsay M. Monte and Hyon B. Shin, "Broad Diversity of Asian, Native Hawaiian, Pacific Islander Population," US Census Bureau, May 25, 2022, https://www.census.gov/library/stories/2022/05/aanhpi-population-diverse-geographically -dispersed.html.

47. P. J. Godolphin et al., "Estimating Interactions and Subgroup-Specific Treatment Effects in Meta-Analysis Without Aggregation Bias: A Within-Trial Framework," *Research Synthesis Methods* 1 (Jan. 14, 2023): 68–78.

48. Stella S. Yi, "Taking Action to Improve Asian American Health," *American Journal of Public Health* 110, no. 4 (2020): 435–37, doi: 10.2105/AJPH.2020 .305596; Jed Keenan Obra et al., "Achieving Equity in Asian American Health-care: Critical Issues and Solutions," *Journal of Asian Health* 1, no. 1 (2021): e202103, doi: 10.59448/jah.v1i1.3.

CHAPTER SEVEN: THE OTHER SIDE

1. "Nahuatl Language," *Encyclopaedia Britannica*, https://www.britannica.com /topic/Nahuatl-language; "Aztec Empire and the Triple Alliance," History.com, https://www.history.com/news/aztec-empire-triple-alliance.

2. Rosa Tupina Yaotonalcuauhtli, interview by Monica Wang, virtual, Boston, MA, May 13, 2022.

3. Kerrie Pickering et al., "Indigenous Peoples and the COVID-19 Pandemic: A Systematic Scoping Review," *Environmental Research Letters* 18, no. 3 (2023): 033001, doi: 10.1088/1748-9326/acb804.

4. Robert Maduro, "Curanderismo and Latino Views of Disease and Curing," *Western Journal of Medicine* 139, no. 6 (1983): 868–74.

5. Benedict I. Truman, Man-Huei Chang, and Ramal Moonesinghe, "Provisional COVID-19 Age-Adjusted Death Rates, by Race and Ethnicity—United States, 2020–2021," *MMWR Morbidity and Mortality Weekly Report* 71, no. 17 (2022): 601–5, doi: 10.15585/mmwr.mm7117e2.

6. Nakari Thorpe, "COVID-19 Cases Are Falling Across NSW but New Infections Emerging in Indigenous Communities," ABC News, Oct. 26, 2021, https://www.abc.net.au/news/2021-10-27/covid-19-cases-still-impacting-indigenous -population/100570000.

7. Nicholas Steyn et al., "Māori and Pacific People in New Zealand Have a Higher Risk of Hospitalisation for COVID-19," *New Zealand Medical Journal* 134, no. 1538 (2021): 28–43.

8. Tamara Power et al., "COVID-19 and Indigenous Peoples: An Imperative for Action," *Journal of Clinical Nursing* 29, nos. 15–16 (2020): 2737–41, doi: 10.1111/jocn.15320.

9. US Centers for Disease Control and Prevention, "Diabetes and American Indians/Alaska Natives," *Healthy People 2020 Database*, 2021, https://minority health.hhs.gov/diabetes-and-american-indiansalaska-natives.

10. US Centers for Disease Control and Prevention, "National Diabetes Statistics Report," May 15, 2024, https://www.cdc.gov/diabetes/php/data-research /index.html.

11. US Department of Health and Human Services, Office of Minority Health, "Obesity and American Indians/Alaska Natives," https://minorityhealth

.hhs.gov/obesity-and-american-indiansalaska-natives#1; National Health Interview Survey, "Table A-15a. Age-Adjusted Percent Distribution (with Standard Errors) of Body Mass Index Among Adults Aged 18 and Over, by Selected Characteristics: United States, 2018," https://www.cdc.gov/nchs/nhis/shs/tables.htm.

12. US Department of Health and Human Services, Office of Minority Health, "Heart Disease and American Indian/Alaska Natives," https://minority health.hhs.gov/heart-disease-and-american-indiansalaska-natives.

13. US Department of Health and Human Services, Office of Minority Health, "Asthma and American Indian/Alaska Natives," https://minorityhealth .hhs.gov/asthma-and-american-indiansalaska-natives.

14. US Centers for Disease Control and Prevention, "Cancer and American Indian and Alaska Native People," Jan. 11, 2024, https://www.cdc.gov/cancer /health-equity/american-indian-alaska-native.html.

15. US Department of Health and Human Services, Indian Health Service, "Disparities," Oct. 2019, https://www.ihs.gov/newsroom/factsheets/disparities/.

16. David S. Jones, "The Persistence of American Indian Health Disparities," *American Journal of Public Health* 96, no. 12 (2006): 2122–34, doi: 10.2105/AJPH .2004.054262.

17. National Academies of Sciences, Engineering, and Medicine; Health and Medicine Division; Board on Population Health and Public Health Practice; Committee on Community-Based Solutions to Promote Health Equity in the United States, A. Baciu et al., eds., *Communities in Action: Pathways to Health Equity* (Washington, DC: National Academies Press, 2017), Appendix A, Native American Health: Historical and Legal Context, https://www.ncbi.nlm.nih.gov/books /NBK425854/.

18. Sunmin Park, Nobuko Hongu, and James Daily III, "Native American Foods: History, Culture, and Influence on Modern Diets," *Journal of Ethnic Foods* 3 (2016), doi: 10.1016/j.jef.2016.08.001.

19. Fred Beauvais, "American Indians and Alcohol," *Alcohol Health & Research World* 22, no. 4 (1998): 253–59.

20. Debra L. Martin and Alan H. Goodman, "Health Conditions Before Columbus: Paleopathology of Native North Americans," *Western Journal of Medicine* 176, no. 1 (2002): 65–68, doi: 10.1136/ewjm.176.1.65.

21. Jamie E. Ehrenpreis and Eli D. Ehrenpreis, "A Historical Perspective of Healthcare Disparity and Infectious Disease in the Native American Population," *American Journal of Medical Sciences* 363, no. 4 (2022): 288–94, doi: 10.1016/j .amjms.2022.01.005.

22. National Libraries of Medicine, "1763–64: Britain Wages Biological Warfare with Smallpox," https://www.nlm.nih.gov/nativevoices/timeline/229.html.

23. David Childs, "Learning from History: Pandemics Are Nothing New in Native Communities," *Democracy and Me*, Apr. 8, 2020, https://www.democracy andme.org/learning-from-history-pandemics-are-nothing-new-in-native -communities/.

24. Libraries of Congress, "Indian Removal Act: Primary Documents in American History," https://guides.loc.gov/indian-removal-act/introduction.

25. National Geographic, "May 28, 1830 CE: Indian Removal Act," https:// education.nationalgeographic.org/resource/indian-removal-act/.

26. Brett Clark, "The Indigenous Environmental Movement in the United States: Transcending Borders in Struggles Against Mining, Manufacturing, and the Capitalist State," *Organization & Environment* 15, no. 4 (2002): 410–42, doi:10.1177/1086026602238170.

27. Michelle Sarche and Paul Spicer, "Poverty and Health Disparities for American Indian and Alaska Native Children: Current Knowledge and Future Prospects," *Annals of the New York Academy of Sciences* 1136 (2008): 126–36, doi: 10.1196/annals.1425.017.

28. Sara U. Maillacheruvu, "The Historic Determinants of Food Insecurity in Native Communities," Center on Budget and Policy Priorities, Oct. 4, 2022, https://www.cbpp.org/research/food-assistance/the-historical-determinants-of -food-insecurity-in-native-communities; "How Native American Diets Shifted After European Colonization," History.com, https://www.history.com/news /native-american-food-shifts.

29. Institute of Medicine (US) Committee on Understanding and Eliminat-ing Racial and Ethnic Disparities in Health Care, Smedley, Brian D., Adrienne Y. Stith, and Alan R. Nelson, eds., *Unequal Treatment: Confronting Racial and Ethnic Disparities in Health Care* (Washington, DC: National Academies Press, 2003).

30. National Archives, "Dawes Act (1887)," https://www.archives.gov/milestone -documents/dawes-act.

31. National Libraries of Medicine, "1934: President Franklin Roosevelt Signs the Indian Reorganization Act," https://www.nlm.nih.gov/nativevoices/timeline /452.html.

32. University of Alaska Fairbanks, "Termination Era, the 1950s, Public Law 280," https://www.uaf.edu/tribal/academics/112/unit-2/terminationerathe1950s publiclaw280.php.

33. Rachel Yehuda and Amy Lehrner, "Intergenerational Transmission of Trauma Effects: Putative Role of Epigenetic Mechanisms," *World Psychiatry* 17, no. 3 (2018): 243–57, doi: 10.1002/wps.20568.

34. Frederick E. Hoxie, *A Final Promise: The Campaign to Assimilate the Indians, 1880–1920* (Lincoln: University of Nebraska Press, 1984); Government of Canada, "First Nations in Canada, Part 4—Legislated Assimilation—Development of the Indian Act (1820–1927)," https://www.rcaanc-cirnac.gc.ca/eng/1307460755710 /1536862806124#chp4; US Department of the Interior, "Federal Indian Boarding School Initiative," doi.gov/priorities/strengthening-indian-country/federal-indian -boarding-school-initiative.

35. Bryan Newland, *Federal Indian Boarding School Initiative Investigative Report*, US Department of the Interior, May 2022, https://www.bia.gov/sites/default/files /dup/inline-files/bsi_investigative_report_may_2022_508.pdf.

36. US Congress. 95th Congress, 2nd Session, House of Representatives, *Report No. 1386: Establishing Standards for the Placement of Indian Children in Foster or Adoptive Homes to Prevent the Breakup of Indian Families, and for Other Purposes*, July 24, 1978, https://www.narf.org/nill/documents/icwa/federal/lh/hr1386.pdf.

37. Kristi Ka'apu and Catherine E. Burnette, "A Culturally Informed Sys-tematic Review of Mental Health Disparities Among Adult Indigenous Men and Women of the USA: What Is Known?" *British Journal of Social Work* 49, no. 4 (2019): 880–98, doi: 10.1093/bjsw/bcz009.

38. Michelle C. Sarche, Paul Spicer, Patricia Farrell, and Hiram E. Fitzgerald, eds., *American Indian and Alaska Native Children and Mental Health: Development, Context, Prevention, and Treatment* (Santa Barbara, CA: Praeger/ABC-CLIO, 2011).

39. Jane Lawrence, "The Indian Health Service and the Sterilization of Native American Women," *American Indian Quarterly* 24, no. 3 (2000): 400–419, doi: 10.1353/aiq.2000.0008; Jennifer Leason, "Forced and Coerced Sterilization of Indigenous Women: Strengths to Build Upon," *Canadian Family Physician* 67, no. 7 (2021): 525–27, doi: 10.46747/cfp.6707525.

40. Neha A. John-Henderson and Annie T. Ginty, "Historical Trauma and Social Support as Predictors of Psychological Stress Responses in American Indian Adults During the COVID-19 Pandemic," *Journal of Psychosomatic Research* 139 (2020): 110263, doi: 10.1016/j.jpsychores.2020.110263.

41. Simon Moya Smith, "Coronavirus Takes More Than Native Americans' Lives. Killing Our Elderly Erases Our Culture," NBC News, Apr. 22, 2020, https://www.nbcnews.com/think/opinion/coronavirus-takes-more-native -americans-lives-killing-our-elderly-erases-ncna1189761; Terri Hansen, "How COVID-19 Could Destroy Indigenous Communities," BBC, July 29, 2020, https://www.bbc.com/future/article/20200727-how-covid-19-could-destroy -indigenous-communities.

42. Ankita Saini, Adya Varshney, Ashok Saini, and Indra Mani, "Insight into Epigenetics and Human Diseases," *Progress in Molecular Biology and Translational Science* 197 (2023): 1–21, doi: 10.1016/bs.pmbts.2023.01.007.

43. Conrad H. Waddington, "The Epigenotype," *Endeavor* 1 (1942): 18–20.

44. Shuk-Mei Ho et al., "Environmental Epigenetics and Its Implication on Disease Risk and Health Outcomes," *ILAR Journal* 53, no. 3–4 (2012): 289–305, doi: 10.1093/ilar.53.3-4.289.

45. US Centers for Disease Control and Prevention, "Epigenetics, Health, and Disease," May 15, 2024, https://www.cdc.gov/genomics-and-health/about /epigenetic-impacts-on-health.html.

46. Louisa M. Villeneuve, Marpadga A. Reddy, and Rama Natarajan, "Epigenetics: Deciphering Its Role in Diabetes and Its Chronic Complications," *Clinical and Experimental Pharmacology and Physiology* 38, no. 7 (2011): 451–59, doi: 10.1111/j.1440-1681.2011.05497.x; Antonella Farsetti, Barbara Illi, and Carlo Gaetano, "How Epigenetics Impacts on Human Diseases," *European Journal of Internal Medicine* 114 (2023): 15–22, doi: 10.1016/j.ejim.2023.05.036.

47. Teresa N. Brockie, Morgan Heinzelmann, and Jessica Gill, "A Framework to Examine the Role of Epigenetics in Health Disparities Among Native Americans," *Nursing Research and Practice* 2013 (2013): 410395, doi: 10.1155/2013/410395; Alexis D. Vick and Heather H. Burris, "Epigenetics and Health Disparities," *Current Epidemiology Reports* 4, no. 1 (2017): 31–37, doi: 10.1007/s40471-017-0096-x.

48. Haoying Wang, "Why the Navajo Nation Was Hit So Hard by Coronavirus: Understanding the Disproportionate Impact of the COVID-19 Pandemic," *Applied Geography* 134 (2021): 102526, doi: 10.1016/j.apgeog.2021.102526.

49. Pearl A. McElfish et al., "COVID-19 Disparities Among Marshallese Pacific Islanders," *Preventing Chronic Disease* 18 (2021): E02, doi: 10.5888/pcd18.200407.

50. US Embassy in the Republic of the Marshall Islands, *The Legacy of U.S. Nuclear Testing and Radiation Exposure in the Marshall Islands*, Sept. 15, 2012,

https://mh.usembassy.gov/the-legacy-of-u-s-nuclear-testing-and-radiation
-exposure-in-the-marshall-islands/; Holly M. Barker, *Bravo for the Marshallese: Regaining Control in a Post-Nuclear World*, 2nd ed. (Cengage Learning, 2012).

51. Harold L. Beck et al., "Fallout Deposition in the Marshall Islands from Bikini and Enewetak Nuclear Weapons Tests," *Health Physics* 99, no. 2 (2010): 124–42, doi: 10.1097/HP.0b013e3181bbbfbd; William Robison, Kenneth Bogen, and Cynthia Conrad, "An Updated Dose Assessment for Resettlement Options at Bikini Atoll—A U.S. Nuclear Test Site," *Health Physics* 73, no. 1 (1997): 100–114, doi: 10.1097/00004032-199707000-00008.

52. Nancy J. Pollock, "Health Transitions, Fast and Nasty: Exposure to Nuclear Radiation," *Pacific Health Dialog* 9, no. 2 (2002): 275–82; Ruth Levy Guyer, "Radioactivity and Rights: Clashes at Bikini Atoll," *American Journal of Public Health* 91, no. 9 (2001): 1371–76, doi: 10.2105/ajph.91.9.1371.

53. US Department of the Interior, *The Compacts of Free Association and Living in the United States*, https://www.doi.gov/oia/COFAinUS.

54. US Congressional Research Service, *The Compacts of Free Association*, updated Apr. 25, 2024, https://crsreports.congress.gov/product/pdf/IF/IF12194.

55. Arkansas Farm Bureau, "Poultry," 2024, https://www.arfb.com/pages /arkansas-agriculture/commodity-corner/poultry/.

56. Pearl McElfish, "Unpublished Preliminary Planning Interviews with Local Marshallese and Marshallese Healthcare Providers from August 2012 Through November 2013," University of Arkansas for Medical Sciences-Northwest, Springdale and Fayetteville, 2012–13.

57. Seiji Yamada et al., "Diabetes Mellitus Prevalence in Out-patient Marshallese Adults on Ebeye Island, Republic of the Marshall Islands," *Hawaii Medical Journal* 63, no. 2 (2004): 45–51; Monica L. Wang et al., "BMI and Related Risk Factors Among U.S. Marshallese with Diabetes and Their Families," *Ethnicity & Health* 26, no. 8 (2021): 1196–1208, doi: 10.1080/13557858.2019 .1640351.

58. Corina S. Penaia, Brittany N. Morey, and Karla B. Thomas, "Disparities in Native Hawaiian and Pacific Islander COVID-19 Mortality: A Community-Driven Data Response," *American Journal of Public Health* 111, no. S2 (2021): S49–S52, doi: 10.2105/AJPH.2021.306370.

59. US Department of Health and Human Services, Office of the Assistant Secretary for Planning and Evaluation, *How Increased Funding Can Advance the Mission of the Indian Health Service to Improve Health Outcomes for American Indians and Alaska Natives* (Report No. HP-2022-21), July 2022, https://aspe.hhs.gov /sites/default/files/documents/e7b3d02affdda1949c215f57b65b5541/aspe-ihs -funding-disparities-report.pdf.

60. US Government Accountability Office, *Indian Health Service: Many Federal Facilities Are in Fair or Poor Condition and Better Data Are Needed on Medical Equipment*, Nov. 2023, https://www.gao.gov/assets/d24105723.pdf.

61. Luz de Atabey, "A Midwifery Project," https://www.lampatx.org/about; Felisa Yzaguirre, interview by Monica Wang, Manchaca, Texas, Nov. 14, 2024.

62. Jeanette W. Schiff and Kerri Moore, "The Impact of the Sweat Lodge Ceremony on Dimensions of Well-Being," *American Indian and Alaska Native Mental Health Research* 13, no. 3 (2006): 48–69, doi:10.5820/aian.1303.2006.48.

63. University of Saskatchewan, "Combating Diabetes Using Community Strengths, Aided by USask Research," Aug. 24, 2023, https://news.usask.ca/articles /research/2023/combating-diabetes-using-community-strengths-aided-by-usask -research.php.

64. Letizia Trevisi et al., "Community Outreach for Navajo People Living with Diabetes: Who Benefits Most?" *Preventing Chronic Disease* 17 (2020): 200068, doi: 10.5888/pcd17.200068.

65. Elizabeth Rink et al., "We Don't Separate Out These Things. Everything Is Related: Partnerships with Indigenous Communities to Design, Implement, and Evaluate Multilevel Interventions to Reduce Health Disparities," *Preventive Science* 25 (Suppl. 3) (2024): 474–85, doi: 10.1007/s11121-024-01668-9.

66. University of Arizona, Cancer Center, "Partnership for Native American Cancer Prevention," https://cancercenter.arizona.edu/researchers/collaborative -research/nacp.

67. Sonya Soni, Jessica Mason, and Jermeen Sherman, "Beyond Human-Centered Design: The Promise of Anti-Racist Community-Centered Approaches in Child Welfare Program and Policy Design," *Child Welfare* 100, no. 1 (2022): 81+.

68. Alaska Native Tribal Health Consortium, 2024, https://www.anthc.org.

CHAPTER EIGHT: DO YOU SEE ME?

1. Gettysburg College, "One Third of Your Life Is Spent at Work," https:// www.gettysburg.edu/news/stories?id=79db7b34-630c-4f49-ad32-4ab9ea48e72b.

2. Robert A. Karasek, "Job Demands, Job Decision Latitude, and Mental Strain: Implications for Job Redesign," *Administrative Science Quarterly* 24, no. 2 (1979): 285–308.

3. Jason Kain and Steve Jex, "Karasek's (1979) Job Demands-Control Model: A Summary of Current Issues and Recommendations for Future Research," in *New Developments in Theoretical and Conceptual Approaches to Job Stress*, ed. P. L. Perrewé and D. C. Ganster (Bingley: Emerald Group Publishing, 2010), 237–68, doi: 10.1108/S1479-3555(2010)0000008009.

4. Robert Karasek and Töres Theorell, *Healthy Work: Stress, Productivity, and the Reconstruction of Working Life* (New York: Basic Books, 1990).

5. Jan Alexander Häusser et al., "Ten Years On: A Review of Recent Research on the Job Demand–Control (-Support) Model and Psychological Well-Being," *Work & Stress* 24, no. 1 (2010): 1–35, doi: 10.1080/02678371003683747; Stephen Stansfeld and Bridget Candy, "Psychosocial Work Environment and Mental Health—A Meta-Analytic Review," *Scandinavian Journal of Work, Environment & Health* 32, no. 6 (2007): 443–62, doi: 10.5271/sjweh.1050; Mika Kivimäki et al., "Work Stress in the Etiology of Coronary Heart Disease—A Meta-Analysis," *Scandinavian Journal of Work, Environment & Health* 32, no. 6 (2006): 431–42, doi: 10.5271/sjweh.1049.

6. Zhuofei Lu et al., "Who Gains Mental Health Benefits from Work Autonomy? The Roles of Gender and Occupational Class," *Applied Research in Quality of Life* (2023): 1–23, doi:10.1007/s11482-023-10161-4; J. A. Landeweerd and N. P. G. Boumans, "The Effect of Work Dimensions and Need for Autonomy on Nurses' Work Satisfaction and Health," *Journal of Occupational and Organizational Psychology* 67 (1994): 207–17, doi: 10.1111/j.2044-8325.1994.tb00563.x; Elise Moreau and Genevieve A. Mageau, "The Importance of Perceived Autonomy

Support for the Psychological Health and Work Satisfaction of Health Professionals: Not Only Supervisors Count, Colleagues Too!" *Motivation and Emotion* 36 (2012): 268–86, doi: 10.1007/s11031-011-9250-9.

7. Sergio Edú-Valsania, Ana Laguía, and Juan A. Moriano, "Burnout: A Review of Theory and Measurement," *International Journal of Environmental Research and Public Health* 19, no. 3 (2022): 1780, doi: 10.3390/ijerph19031780.

8. World Health Organization, "Burnout—an 'Occupational Phenomenon': International Classification of Diseases," May 28, 2019, https://www.who.int/news/item/28-05-2019-burn-out-an-occupational-phenomenon-international-classification-of-diseases.

9. GBAO, "Healthcare Workers: Poll Analysis," Dec. 13, 2021, https://static1.squarespace.com/static/619c009fb3e63b1bb3d3684f/t/61b781ef3825d3535437a6e5/1639416303381/Healthcare+Workers+Memo+121321.pdf.

10. Crown Counseling, "15+ Social Work Burnout Statistics," https://crowncounseling.com/statistics/social-worker-burnout-statistics/.

11. Gallup, "K-12 Workers Have Highest Burnout Rate in the U.S.," June 13, 2021, https://news.gallup.com/poll/393500/workers-highest-burnout-rate.aspx.

12. Future Forum, "Future Forum Pulse," Feb. 2023, https://futureforum.com/research/future-forum-pulse-winter-2022-2023-snapshot/#what-percentage-of-the-workforce-is-burned-out.

13. Jourdyn A. Lawrence et al., "Racial/Ethnic Differences in Burnout: A Systematic Review," *Journal of Racial and Ethnic Health Disparities* 9, no. 1 (2022): 257–69, doi: 10.1007/s40615-020-00950-0.

14. Jessica Shakesprere, Batia Katz, and Pamela Loprest, "Racial Equity and Job Quality Causes Behind Racial Disparities and Possibilities to Address Them," Urban Institute, September 2021, https://www.urban.org/sites/default/files/publication/104761/racial-equity-and-job-quality.pdf.

15. Robin Bleiweis, Jocelyn Frye, and Rose Khattar, "Women of Color and the Wage Gap," Center for American Progress, Nov. 17, 2021, https://www.americanprogress.org/article/women-of-color-and-the-wage-gap/.

16. "Women in the Workplace 2023," McKinsey & Company, https://sgff-media.s3.amazonaws.com/sgff_r1eHetbDYb/Women+in+the+Workplace+2023_+Designed+Report.pdf; Katherine Haan, "Gender Pay Gap Statistics," *Forbes*, updated Mar. 1, 2024, https://www.forbes.com/advisor/business/gender-pay-gap-statistics/; Heejung Chung and Tanja van der Lippe, "Flexible Working, Work-Life Balance, and Gender Equality: Introduction," *Social Indicators Research* 151 (2020): 365–81, doi: 10.1007/s11205-018-2025-x.

17. Lisa Huynh, "Employment Barriers within Low and Moderate-Income Communities," US Bureau of Labor Statistics, Mar. 2020, https://www.bls.gov/opub/mlr/2020/beyond-bls/employment-barriers-within-low-and-moderate-income-communities.htm; André Dua et al., "Freelance, Side Hustles, and Gigs: Many More Americans Have Become Independent Workers," McKinsey & Company, Aug. 23, 2022, https://www.mckinsey.com/featured-insights/sustainable-inclusive-growth/future-of-america/freelance-side-hustles-and-gigs-many-more-americans-have-become-independent-workers; "Freelance Forward 2023 Research Report," Upwork, Dec. 12, 2023, https://www.upwork.com/research/freelance-forward-2023-research-report.

18. Analysts of the National Estimates Branch, "Current Employment Statistics Highlights," US Bureau of Labor Statistics, Dec. 2024, https://www.bls.gov /web/empsit/ceshighlights.pdf; "Staffing Employment Declined in First Quarter of 2024," American Staffing Association, June 27, 2024, https://americanstaffing.net /posts/2024/06/27/staffing-employment-declined-in-first-quarter-of-2024/.

19. Ibraheem S. Al-Tarawneh, Steven J. Wurzelbacher, and Stephen J. Bertke, "Comparative Analysis of Workers' Compensation Claims of Injury Among Temporary and Permanent Employed Workers in Ohio," *American Journal of Industrial Medicine* (2019): 1–20, doi: 10.1002/ajim.23049; Michael Foley, "Factors Underlying Observed Injury Rate Differences Between Temporary Workers and Permanent Peers," *American Journal of Industrial Medicine* 60, no. 10 (2017): 841–51, doi: 10.1002/ajim.22763.

20. "Temporary Jobs Growing Fast, Temp Workers Legal Protections," National Employment Law Project, Aug. 26, 2019, https://www.nelp.org/news-release /temporary-jobs-growing-fast-temp-workers-legal-protections/.

21. Tae Jun Kim and Olaf von dem Knesebeck, "Is an Insecure Job Better for Health Than Having No Job at All? A Systematic Review of Studies Investigating the Health-Related Risks of Both Job Insecurity and Unemployment," *BMC Public Health* 15 (2015): 985, doi: 10.1186/s12889-015-2313-1.

22. Paul A. Landsbergis, Joseph G. Grzywacz, and Anthony D. LaMontagne, "Work Organization, Job Insecurity, and Occupational Health Disparities," *American Journal of Industrial Medicine* 57, no. 5 (2014): 495–515, doi: 10.1002/ajim.22126.

23. H. De Witte, "On the Scarring Effects of Job Insecurity (and How They Can Be Explained)," *Scandinavian Journal of Work, Environment & Health* 42, no. 2 (2016): 99–102, doi: 10.5271/sjweh.3545.

24. Jagdish Khubchandani and James Price, "Association of Job Insecurity with Health Risk Factors and Poorer Health in American Workers," *Journal of Community Health* 42, no. 2 (2017): 242–51, doi: 10.1007/s10900-016-0249-8.

25. Abida Ayub, Mehwish Majeed, and Rabia Imran, "Impact of Organizational Justice, Job Security and Job Satisfaction on Organizational Productivity," *Journal of Economics, Business and Management* 3 (2015), doi:10.7763/JOEBM.2015.V3.295.

26. Lixin Jiang, Amy Lawrence, and Xiaohong Violet Xu, "Does a Stick Work? A Meta-Analytic Examination of Curvilinear Relationships Between Job Insecurity and Employee Workplace Behaviors," *Journal of Organizational Behavior* 43 (2022), doi:10.1002/job.2652.

27. Philip Whyman and Alina Petrescu, "Workplace Flexibility Practices in SMEs: Relationship with Performance via Redundancies, Absenteeism, and Financial Turnover," *Journal of Small Business Management* 53, no. 4 (2015): 1097–1126, doi: 10.1111/jsbm.12092.

28. Monica L. Wang et al., "Job Flexibility, Job Security, and Mental Health Among US Working Adults," *JAMA Network Open* 7, no. 3 (2024): e243439, doi:10.1001/jamanetworkopen.2024.3439.

29. Rahman Shiri et al., "The Effect of Employee-Oriented Flexible Work on Mental Health: A Systematic Review," *Healthcare* 10, no. 5 (2022): 883, doi: 10.3390/healthcare10050883.

30. Monica L. Wang et al., "Gender Disparities in Job Flexibility, Job Security, Psychological Distress, Work Absenteeism, and Work Presenteeism among U.S.

Adults," *Social Science Medicine Population Health* 29 (2025): 101761, doi: 10.1016/j
.ssmph.2025.101761.

31. Gizelda Rodrigues de Araújo, Josiane Machado Fagundes Freitas, and
Nayara Aryan Melo Souza, "The Historical Role of Women's Insertion in the
Labor Market and Their Double Shift," *Revista Científica Multidisciplinar Núcleo do
Conhecimento* 11, no. 4 (2021): 76-97, doi: 10.32749/nucleodoconhecimento.com
br/history/womens-insertion.

32. Sarah M. Flood et al., "American Time Use Survey Data Extract Builder:
Version 3.2," in *American Time Use Survey 2023* (College Park: University of
Maryland: IPUMS, 2023), doi: 10.18128/D060.V3.2.

33. Soraya Seedat and Marta Rondon, "Women's Wellbeing and the Burden of
Unpaid Work," *Lancet* 374 (2021): n1972, doi: 10.1136/bmj.n1972.

34. Chloe E. Bird, "Gender, Household Labor, and Psychological Distress:
The Impact of the Amount and Division of Housework," *Journal of Health and
Social Behavior* 40, no. 1 (1999): 32–45.

35. Paraskevi Peristera, Hugo Westerlund, and Linda L. Magnusson Han-
son, "Paid and Unpaid Working Hours Among Swedish Men and Women in
Relation to Depressive Symptom Trajectories: Results from Four Waves of the
Swedish Longitudinal Occupational Survey of Health," *BMJ Open* 8 (2018):
e017525, doi: 10.1136/bmjopen-2017-017525; Irene Magaña, Pablo Martínez,
and Maria Soledad Loyola, "Health Outcomes of Unpaid Caregivers in Low- and
Middle-Income Countries: A Systematic Review and Meta-Analysis," *Journal of
Clinical Nursing* 29 (2020): 3950–65, doi: 10.1111/jocn.15450.

36. Lisa M. Dinella et al., "Women Disproportionately Shoulder Burdens
Imposed by the Global COVID-19 Pandemic," *Journal of Social Issues* 79 (2023):
1057–87, doi: 10.1111/josi.12591.

37. "Whose Time to Care? Unpaid Care and Domestic Work During
COVID-19," UN Women, https://data.unwomen.org/sites/default/files/inline
-files/Whose-time-to-care-brief_0.pdf.

38. Mark Wade et al., "The Disparate Impact of COVID-19 on the Mental
Health of Female and Male Caregivers," *Social Science & Medicine* 275 (2021):
113801, doi: 10.1016/j.socscimed.2021.113801.

39. Theresa M. Bastain et al., "COVID-19 Pandemic Experiences and Symptoms
of Pandemic-Associated Traumatic Stress Among Mothers in the US," *JAMA Network Open* 5, no. 12 (2022): e2247330, doi:10.1001/jamanetworkopen.2022.47330.

40. Sandrine Lungumbu and Amelia Butterly, "Coronavirus and Gender:
More Chores for Women Set Back Gains in Equality," BBC, Nov. 25, 2020,
https://www.bbc.com/news/world-55016842.

41. Michele Berger, "How Have Women in the Workforce Fared, Three Years
into the Pandemic?" *Penn Today*, Mar. 20, 2023, https://penntoday.upenn.edu/news
/how-have-women-workforce-fared-three-years-pandemic.

42. Arlie Russell Hochschild and Anne Machung, *The Second Shift: Working
Parents and the Revolution At Home* (New York: Viking, 1989).

43. Samantha Ndiwalana, "It's a Man's World: Men Still Dominate the Most
Influential Companies in the World," World Benchmarking Alliance, Sept. 30,
2020, https://www.worldbenchmarkingalliance.org/news/its-a-mans-world-men
-still-dominate-the-most-influential-companies-in-the-world/.

44. Beniamino Cislaghi et al., "Gender Norms and Gender Equality in Full-Time Employment and Health: A 97-Country Analysis of the World Values Survey," *Frontiers in Psychology* 13 (2022): 689815, doi: 10.3389/fpsyg.2022.689815.

45. "America at Work," Library of Congress, https://www.loc.gov/collections/america-at-work-and-leisure-1894-to-1915/articles-and-essays/america-at-work/.

46. Janet L. Yellen, "The History of Women's Work and Wages and How It Has Created Success for Us All," *Brookings*, May 2020, https://www.brookings.edu/articles/the-history-of-womens-work-and-wages-and-how-it-has-created-success-for-us-all/.

47. Jonathan Grossman, "Fair Labor Standards Act of 1938: Maximum Struggle for a Minimum Wage," US Department of Labor, https://www.dol.gov/general/aboutdol/history/flsa1938.

48. Katherine Eyster, "Fighting for Fairness: Domestic Workers and the Fair Labor Standards Act," *US Department of Labor Blog*, Apr. 12, 2024, https://blog.dol.gov/2024/04/12/fighting-for-fairness-domestic-workers-and-the-fair-labor-standards-act.

49. Mildred A. Joiner and Clarence M. Weiner, "Employment of Women in War Production," *Social Security Bulletin* 5, no. 7 (1942): 4–15, https://www.ssa.gov/policy/docs/ssb/v5n7/v5n7p4.pdf; National Park Service, *World War II and the American Home Front*, https://www.nps.gov/articles/000/the-american-home-front-and-world-war-ii.htm.

50. PBS, "Women and Work After World War II," https://www.pbs.org/wgbh/americanexperience/features/tupperware-work/.

51. Sarah Pruitt, "The Post World War II Boom: How America Got into Gear," History.com, updated Aug. 10, 2023, originally published May 14, 2020, https://www.history.com/news/post-world-war-ii-boom-economy.

52. Jessica Schieder and Elise Gould, *"Women's Work" and the Gender Pay Gap: How Discrimination, Societal Norms, and Other Forces Affect Women's Occupational Choices—and Their Pay*, Economic Policy Institute, July 20, 2016, https://www.epi.org/publication/womens-work-and-the-gender-pay-gap-how-discrimination-societal-norms-and-other-forces-affect-womens-occupational-choices-and-their-pay/.

53. Amy Heshmati, Helena Honkaniemi, and Sol P. Juárez, "The Effect of Parental Leave on Parents' Mental Health: A Systematic Review," *Lancet Public Health* 8, no. 1 (2023): e57–e75; Mariam S. Khan, "Paid Family Leave and Children Health Outcomes in OECD Countries," *Child and Youth Services Review* 116 (2020): 105259, doi: 10.1016/j.childyouth; Maureen Sayres Van Niel et al., "The Impact of Paid Maternity Leave on the Mental and Physical Health of Mothers and Children: A Review of the Literature and Policy Implications," *Harvard Review of Psychiatry* 28, no. 2 (2020): 113–26, doi: 10.1097/HRP.0000000000000246.

54. US Department of Labor, "The Family and Medical Leave Act of 1993," https://www.dol.gov/agencies/whd/laws-and-regulations/laws/fmla.

55. The White House, "On Anniversary of Equal Pay Act, Signs of Progress and Remaining Challenges for Women in the Labor Market," June 21, 2023, https://www.whitehouse.gov/cea/written-materials/2023/06/21/on-anniversary-of-equal-pay-act-signs-of-progress-and-remaining-challenges-for-women-in-the-labor-market/.

56. Adam Burtle and Stephen Bezruchka, "Population Health and Paid Parental Leave: What the United States Can Learn from Two Decades of Research," *Healthcare* 4, no. 2 (2016): 30. doi: 10.3390/healthcare4020030; Ann Bartel et al., "The Impacts of Paid Family and Medical Leave on Worker Health, Family Well-Being, and Employer Outcomes," *Annual Review of Public Health* 44 (2023): 429–43, doi: 10.1146/annurev-publhealth-071521-025257.

57. Willem Adema et al., "Paid Parental Leave: Big Differences for Mothers and Fathers," Organization for Economic Cooperation and Development (OECD) Statistics, Jan. 12, 2023, https://oecdstatistics.blog/2023/01/12/paid -parental-leave-big-differences-for-mothers-and-fathers/.

58. Nordic Co-operation, "Parental Benefit in Sweden," https://www.norden .org/en/info-norden/parental-benefit-sweden.

59. Norway, European Commission, Employment, Social Affairs, and Inclusion: Policies and Activities," https://ec.europa.eu/social/main.jsp?catId=1123 &intPageId=4704&langId=en#.

60. InfoFinland, "Holidays and Leaves in Finland," Aug. 14, 2024, https:// www.infofinland.fi/en/work-and-enterprise/during-employment/holidays-and -leaves#heading-804deca7-74f8-4f2e-a46a-dacd7c1c406d.

61. Ásdís Aðalbjörg Arnalds, Guðný Björk Eydal, and Ingólfur V. Gíslason, "Paid Parental Leave in Iceland: Increasing Gender Equality at Home and on the Labour Market," in *Successful Public Policy in the Nordic Countries: Cases, Lessons, Challenges*, ed. Caroline de la Porte et al. (Oxford: Oxford Academic, 2022); Nordic Co-operation, "Maternity/Paternity Leave in Iceland," https://www.norden .org/en/info-norden/maternitypaternity-leave-iceland.

62. US Department of Health and Human Services, *Parents Under Pressure: The U.S. Surgeon General's Advisory on the Mental Health & Well-Being of Parents*, 2024, https://www.hhs.gov/sites/default/files/parents-under-pressure.pdf.

63. Karina Monesson, "4 Actionable Strategies for Achieving Pay Equity," UKG, Mar. 12, 2024, https://www.ukg.com/blog/hr/4-actionable-strategies-achieving-pay -equity; Marie Hatter, "How to Improve Pay Equity at Your Company," *Forbes*, Nov. 17, 2023, https://www.forbes.com/councils/forbescommunicationscouncil/2023/11 /17/how-to-improve-pay-equity-at-your-company/.

64. Tapas K. Ray and Regina Pana-Cryan, "Work Flexibility and Work-Related Well-Being," *International Journal of Environmental Research and Public Health* 18, no. 6 (2021): 3254, doi: 10.3390/ijerph18063254; Sheshadri Chatterjee, Ranjan Chaudhuri, and Demetris Vrontis, "Does Remote Work Flexibility Enhance Organization Performance? The Moderating Role of Organization Policy and Top Management Support," *Journal of Business Research* 139 (2022): 1501–12, doi: 10.1016/j.jbusres .2021.10.069.

65. Lin Rouvroye et al., "Employers' Views on Flexible Employment Contracts for Younger Workers: Benefits, Downsides, and Societal Outlook," *Economic and Industrial Democracy* 43, no. 4 (2021): 1934–57, doi: 10.1177/0143831X211053378; T. J. Kim and O. von dem Knesebeck, "Perceived Job Insecurity, Unemployment, and Depressive Symptoms: A Systematic Review and Meta-Analysis of Prospective Observational Studies," *International Archives of Occupational and Environmental Health* 89, no. 4 (2016): 561–73, doi: 10.1007/s00420-015-1107-1.

66. Alexis Krivkovich, Emily Field, Lareina Yee, and Megan McConnell, with Hannah Smith, *Women in the Workplace 2024: The 10th-Anniversary Report*, McKinsey and Company, Sept. 17, 2024, https://www.mckinsey.com/featured -insights/diversity-and-inclusion/women-in-the-workplace.

67. Care.com Editorial Staff, "This Is How Much Child Care Costs in 2024?" Care.com, Jan. 17, 2024, https://www.care.com/c/how-much-does-child-care-cost/; United Way NCA, "Childcare Cost Burden for Low-Income Households in the U.S.," Oct. 14, 2023, https://unitedwaynca.org/blog/childcare-cost-burden-for-low -income-households-in-the-us/.

68. The White House, "Child Tax Credit," https://www.whitehouse.gov/child -tax-credit/.

69. Isabela Salas-Betsch, "Universal Paid Sick Time Would Strengthen Public Health and Benefit Businesses," Center for American Progress, May 15, 2023, https://www.americanprogress.org/article/universal-paid-sick-time-would -strengthen-public-health-and-benefit-businesses/.

CHAPTER NINE: THE LIGHT IN THE DARK

1. Elizabeth Nix, "Tuskegee Experiment: The Infamous Syphilis Study," History.com, May 16, 2017, updated June 13, 2023, https://www.history.com/news /the-infamous-40-year-tuskegee-study.

2. Stephen B. Thomas and Sandra C. Quinn, "The Tuskegee Syphilis Study, 1932 to 1972: Implications for HIV Education and AIDS Risk Education Programs in the Black Community," *American Journal of Public Health* 81, no. 11 (1991): 1498–1505, doi: 10.2105/ajph.81.11.1498.

3. Robert M. White, "Misinformation and Misbeliefs in the Tuskegee Study of Untreated Syphilis Fuel Mistrust in the Healthcare System," *National Medical Association* 97, no. 11 (2005): 1566–73.

4. COVID Tracking Project, "The COVID Racial Data Tracker," https:// covidtracking.com/race.

5. US Centers for Disease Control and Prevention, "COVID-19 Vaccine Uptake and CDC's Commitment to Vaccine Equity," Nov. 22, 2023, https://www .cdc.gov/ncird/whats-new/vaccine-equity.html.

6. USA Facts, "Alabama Coronavirus Vaccination Progress," https://usafacts .org/visualizations/covid-vaccine-tracker-states/state/alabama/.

7. Yasmine AlSayyad, "An Alabama Woman's Neighborly Vaccination Campaign," *New Yorker*, Aug. 11, 2021, https://www.newyorker.com/culture/the-new-yorker -documentary/an-alabama-womans-neighborly-vaccination-campaign.

8. USA Today Network Ventures Staff, "Alabama's Dorothy Oliver Named Best of Womankind, Gets Special Nod from Dr. Fauci, During USA TODAY's Best of Humankind Awards," *USA Today*, Dec. 9, 2021, https://www.usatoday.com /story/life/humankind/2021/12/09/alabamas-dorothy-oliver-wins-best-humankind -award-vaccination-effort/8889803002/.

9. Cheryl Merzel and Joanna D'Afflitti, "Reconsidering Community-Based Health Promotion: Promise, Performance, and Potential," *American Journal of Public Health* 93 (2003): 557–74, doi: 10.2105/ajph.93.4.557; United Way NCA, "Childcare Cost Burden for Low-Income Households in the U.S.," Oct. 14, 2023,

https://unitedwaynca.org/blog/childcare-cost-burden-for-low-income-households-in-the-us/.

10. Alison O'Mara-Eves et al., "The Effectiveness of Community Engagement in Public Health Interventions for Disadvantaged Groups: A Meta-Analysis," *BMC Public Health* 15 (2015): 129, doi: 10.1186/s12889-015-1352-y.

11. Kasim Ortiz et al., "Partnerships, Processes, and Outcomes: A Health Equity-Focused Scoping Meta-Review of Community-Engaged Scholarship," *Annual Review of Public Health* 41 (2020): 177–99, doi: 10.1146/annurev-publhealth-040119-094220.

12. Darcy Jones McMaughan et al., "Promoting and Advocating for Ethical Community Engagement: Transparency in the Community-engaged Research Spectrum," *Progress in Community Health Partnerships: Research, Education, and Action* 15, no. 4 (2021): 419–24, doi: 10.1353/cpr.2021.0054.

13. Sheila Cyril et al., "Exploring the Role of Community Engagement in Improving the Health of Disadvantaged Populations: A Systematic Review," *Global Health Action* 8 (2015): 29842, doi: 10.3402/gha.v8.29842.

14. Dorothea S. von Goeler et al., "Self-Management of Type 2 Diabetes: A Survey of Low-Income Urban Puerto Ricans," *Diabetes Educator* 29, no. 4 (2003): 663–72, doi: 10.1177/014572170302900412; Milagros C. Rosal et al., "Views and Preferences of Low-Literate Hispanics Regarding Diabetes Education: Results of Formative Research," *Health Education & Behavior* 31, no. 3 (2004): 388–405, doi: 10.1177/1090198104263360; Elena T. Carbone et al., "Diabetes Self-Management: Perspectives of Latino Patients and Their Health Care Providers," *Patient Education and Counseling* 66, no. 2 (2007): 202–10, doi: 10.1016/j.pec.2006.12.003.

15. Milagros C. Rosal et al., "Design and Methods for a Randomized Clinical Trial of a Diabetes Self-Management Intervention for Low-Income Latinos: Latinos en Control," *BMC Medical Research Methodology* 9 (2009): 81, doi: 10.1186/1471-2288-9-81.

16. Milagros C. Rosal et al., "Randomized Trial of a Literacy-Sensitive, Culturally Tailored Diabetes Self-Management Intervention for Low-Income Latinos: Latinos en Control," *Diabetes Care* 34, no. 4 (2011): 838–44, doi: 10.2337/dc10-1981; Monica L. Wang et al., "Who Benefits from Diabetes Self-Management Interventions? The Influence of Depression in the Latinos en Control Trial," *Annals of Behavioral Medicine* 48, no. 2 (2014): 256–64, doi: 10.1007/s12160-014-9606-y.

17. P. G. Sepsis et al., "Seniors' Ratings of the Helpfulness of Health Promotion Features in Starting and Maintaining Physical Activity," *Journal of Aging and Physical Activity* 3 (1995): 193–207; Kristin M. Mills et al., "Consideration of Older Adults' Preferences for Format of Physical Activity," *Journal of Aging and Physical Activity* 5 (1997): 50–58, doi.org/10.1123/japa.5.1.50; Anita L. Stewart et al., "Evaluation of CHAMPS, a Physical Activity Promotion Program for Older Adults," *Annals of Behavioral Medicine* 19 (1997): 353–61, doi: 10.1007/BF02895154.

18. Anita L. Stewart, "Community-Based Physical Activity Programs for Adults Aged 50 and Older," *Journal of Aging and Physical Activity* 9 (2001): S71–S91; Anita L. Stewart et al., "Physical Activity Outcomes of CHAMPS II: A

Physical Activity Promotion Program for Older Adults," *Journal of Gerontology: Biological Sciences* 56, no. 8 (2001): M465–M470, doi: 10.1093/gerona/56.8 .m465; Anita L. Stewart et al., "The California Active Aging Community Grant Program: Translating Science into Practice to Promote Physical Activity in Older Adults," *Annals of Behavioral Medicine* 29, no. 3 (2005): 155–65, doi: 10 .1207/s15324796abm2903_1; Hilary K. Seligman et al., "Improving Physical Activity Resource Guides to Bridge the Divide Between the Clinic and the Community," *Preventing Chronic Disease* 6, no. 1 (2009): A18; Anita L. Stewart et al., "Diffusing a Research-Based Physical Activity Promotion Program for Seniors into Diverse Communities: CHAMPS III," *Preventing Chronic Disease* 3, no. 2 (2006): A51.

19. Gary H. Gibbons and Eliseo J. Pérez-Stable, "Harnessing the Power of Community-Engaged Research," *American Journal of Public Health* 114, no. S1 (2024): S7–S11, doi: 10.2105/AJPH.2023.307528.

20. National Institutes of Health, National Heart, Blood, and Lung Institute Roundtable, "COVID-19 Community-Engaged Research," July 10, 2020, https://www.nhlbi.nih.gov/events/2020/covid-19-community-engaged-research-roundtable.

21. National Institutes of Health, Community Engagement Alliance, "The Power of Listening," May 7, 2021, https://nihceal.org/news/power-of-listening.

22. National Institutes of Health, Community Engagement Alliance, "Animated Video Aims to Increase Trial Participation Among Communities of Color," Mar. 7, 2022, https://nihceal.org/news/animated-video-aims-increase-trial-participation-among-communities-of-color.

23. National Institutes of Health, Community Engagement Alliance, "The Secret to Boosting Vaccine Confidence? It Comes from the Community," July 7, 2021, https://nihceal.org/news/secret-boosting-vaccine-confidence-it-comes-community.

24. South Dakota News, "Brookings Community Pilots Breastfeeding Business Initiative," Mar. 22, 2016, https://news.sd.gov/news?id=news_kb_article_view &sys_id=6e4bd18c1b1c69506e4aa97ae54bcbe6.

25. Jenn Anderson et al., "Brookings Supports Breastfeeding: Using Public Deliberation as a Community-Engaged Approach to Dissemination of Research," *Translational Behavioral Medicine* 7, no. 4 (2017): 783–92, doi: 10.1007/s13142-017 -0480-6.

26. Marc A. Zimmerman et al., "Youth Empowerment Solutions: Evaluation of an After-School Program to Engage Middle School Students in Community Change," *Health Education and Behavior* 45, no. 1 (2018): 20–31, doi: 10.1177 /1090198117710491.

27. Marc A. Zimmerman, "Empowerment Theory," in *Handbook of Community Psychology*, ed. J. Rappaport and E. Seidman (New York: Springer, 2000), 43–63.

28. Local Trust, "About Big Local," https://localtrust.org.uk/big-local/about -big-local/.

29. J. Popay et al., "The Communities in Control Study," *Investigating Health and Social Outcomes of the Big Local Community Empowerment Initiative in England: A Mixed Method Evaluation*, National Institute for Health and Care Research,

2023 (Public Health Research, No. 11.09), https://www.ncbi.nlm.nih.gov/books/NBK597409/.

30. Deanna Kerrigan et al., "A Community Empowerment Approach to the HIV Response among Sex Workers: Effectiveness, Challenges, and Considerations for Implementation and Scale-Up," *Lancet* 385, no. 9963 (2015): 172–85, doi: 10.1016/S0140-6736(14)60973-9.

31. Deanna L. Kerrigan et al., "Community Empowerment among Sex Workers Is an Effective HIV Prevention Intervention: A Systematic Review of the Peer-Reviewed Evidence from Low- and Middle-Income Countries," *AIDS and Behavior* 17, no. 6 (2013): 1926–40, doi: 10.1007/s10461-013-0458-4.

32. Lisa Wexler et al., "Promoting Positive Youth Development and Highlighting Reasons for Living in Northwest Alaska Through Digital Storytelling," *Health Promotion Practice* 14 (2013): 617–23, doi: 10.1177/1524839912462390; Linda Sprague Martinez et al., "Engaging Youth of Color in Applied Science Education and Public Health Promotion," *International Journal of Science Education* 38, no. 4 (2016): 688–99, doi: 10.1080/09500693.2015.1134850; Elizabeth A. Rogers et al., "Engaging Minority Youth in Diabetes Prevention Efforts through a Participatory, Spoken-Word Social Marketing Campaign," *American Journal of Health Promotion* 31, no. 4 (2017): 336–39, doi: 10.4278/ajhp.141215-ARB-624.

33. Monica L. Wang et al., "Design and Methods for a Community-Based Intervention to Reduce Sugar-Sweetened Beverage Consumption among Youth: H2GO! Study," *BMC Public Health* 16, no. 1 (2016): 1150, doi: 10.1186/s12889-016-3803-5; Monica L. Wang et al., "A Youth Empowerment Intervention to Prevent Childhood Obesity: Design and Methods for a Cluster Randomized Trial of the H2GO! Program," *BMC Public Health* 21, no. 1 (2021): 1675, doi: 10.1186/s12889-021-11660-5.

34. Monica L. Wang et al., "Reducing Sugary Drink Intake Through Youth Empowerment: Results from a Pilot-Site Randomized Study," *International Journal of Behavioral Nutrition and Physical Activity* 16, no. 1 (2019): 58, doi: 10.1186/s12966-019-0819-0.

35. Nina Wallerstein, Bonnie Duran, John G. Oetzel, and Meredith Minkler, eds., *Community-Based Participatory Research for Health*, 3rd ed. (San Francisco: Jossey-Bass, 2017).

36. Nina Wallerstein and Bonnie Duran, "Using Community-Based Participatory Research to Address Health Disparities," *Health Promotion Practice* 7 (2006): 312–23, doi: 10.1177/1524839906289376.

37. Jennifer A. Campbell, Alice Yan, and Leonard E. Egede, "Community-Based Participatory Research Interventions to Improve Diabetes Outcomes: A Systematic Review," *Diabetes Educator* 46, no. 6 (2020): 527–39, doi: 10.1177/0145721720962969.

38. Center for American Indian Health Research, Hudson College of Public Health, "Strong Heart Study," University of Oklahoma Health Sciences Center, https://strongheartstudy.org.

39. Kate Stringer, "How Partnerships between Tribal Communities and Researchers like Mandy Fretts Are Improving Heart Health," *University of Washington School of Public Health News*, Nov. 30, 2022, https://epi.washington.edu/news

/how-partnerships-between-tribal-communities-and-researchers-like-mandy
-fretts-are-improving-heart-health/.

40. Center for American Indian Health Research, Hudson College of Public
Health, "Strong Heart Study Publications," University of Oklahoma Health Sci-
ences Center, https://strongheartstudy.org/Research/Papers-and-Abstracts
/Published-Papers#383291822-papers-in-print-in-order-of-year-published.

41. California State University, Fullerton, "Weaving an Islander Network for
Cancer Awareness, Research, and Training (WINCART)," http://wincart.fullerton
.edu/index.htm.

42. Paula Healani Palmer et al., "Eliminating Tobacco Disparities Among
Native Hawaiian Pacific Islanders Through Policy Change: The Role of
Community-Based Organizations," *Health Promotion Practice* 14, no. 5 Suppl.
(2013): 36S–39S, doi: 10.1177/1524839913486150; Paula H. Palmer, "Improv-
ing Pacific Islander Health Through Community Participation: A Case Study,"
in *Health Promotion in Multicultural Populations*, ed. R. M. Huff, M. V. Kline,
and D. V. Peterson (Thousand Oaks, CA: SAGE Publications, 2014), 425–34;
S. P. Tanjasiri et al., "Developing a Community-Based Collaboration to Reduce
Cancer Health Disparities Among Pacific Islanders in California," *Pacific Health
Dialog* 14, no. 1 (2007): 119–27; Mandy LaBreche et al., "Let's Move for Pacific
Islander Communities: An Evidence-Based Intervention to Increase Physical
Activity," *Journal of Cancer Education* 31, no. 2 (2016): 261–67, doi: 10.1007
/s13187-015-0875-3.

43. Kaiser Permanente, Community Health, "HEAL and HEAL Zones,"
https://community.kp.org/about/program/heal-zones.

44. Allen Cheadle et al., "A Community-Level Initiative to Prevent Obesity:
Results from Kaiser Permanente's Healthy Eating Active Living Zones Initiative
in California," *American Journal of Preventive Medicine* 54, no. 5 Suppl. 2 (2018):
S150–S159, doi: 10.1016/j.amepre.2018.01.024.

45. Robert Wood Johnson Foundation, "RWJF Culture of Health Prize:
Communities Leading the Way," 2023, https://www.rwjf.org/en/grants/grantee
-stories/culture-of-health-prize.html.

46. Robert Wood Johnson Foundation, "Austin, Texas: 2023 RWJF Culture
of Health Prize Winner," 2023, https://www.rwjf.org/content/rwjf-web/us/en
/grants/grantee-stories/2023/2023-winner-austin-tx.html; Robert Wood Johnson
Foundation, "Detroit, Michigan: 2023 RWJF Culture of Health Prize Winner,"
2023, https://www.rwjf.org/content/rwjf-web/us/en/grants/grantee-stories/2023
/2023-winner-detroit-mi.html.

47. Robert Wood Johnson Foundation, "Fond du Lac Band of Lake Superior
Chippewa Reservation: 2023 RWJF Culture of Health Prize Winner," https://
www.rwjf.org/content/rwjf-web/us/en/grants/grantee-stories/2023/2023-winner
-fond-du-lac-band-of-lake-superior-chippewa-reservation.html.

CHAPTER TEN: THE COLLECTIVE CURE

1. Blue Zones, "About Blue Zones," https://www.bluezones.com.

2. Dan Buettner, *The Blue Zones: 9 Lessons for Living Longer from the People
Who've Lived the Longest*, 2nd ed. (Washington, DC: National Geographic, 2012).

3. Dan Buettner and Sam Skemp, "Blue Zones: Lessons From the World's Longest Lived," *American Journal of Lifestyle Medicine* 10, no. 5 (2016): 318–21, doi: 10.1177/1559827616637066.

4. Michel Poulain, Anne Herm, and Gianne Pes, "The Blue Zones: Areas of Exceptional Longevity Around the World," *Vienna Yearbook of Population Research* 11 (2013): 87–108.

5. D. Craig Willcox et al., "The Cultural Context of 'Successful Aging' Among Older Women Weavers in a Northern Okinawan Village: The Role of Productive Activity," *Journal of Cross-Cultural Gerontology* 22, no. 2 (2007): 137–65, doi: 10.1007/s10823-006-9032-0.

6. Gianni Pes et al., "Lifestyle and Nutrition Related to Male Longevity in Sardinia: An Ecological Study," *Nutrition, Metabolism, and Cardiovascular Diseases* 23, no. 3 (2013): 212–19, doi: 10.1016/j.numecd.2011.05.004.

7. Romain Legrand et al., "Description of Lifestyle, Including Social Life, Diet, and Physical Activity, of People ≥90 Years Living in Ikaria, a Longevity Blue Zone," *International Journal of Environmental Research and Public Health* 18, no. 12 (2021): 6602, doi: 10.3390/ijerph18126602.

8. Blue Zones, Blue Zones Project Services, https://www.bluezones.com /services/blue-zones-project/#section-2.

9. Blue Zones, "Blue Zones Approach," https://www.bluezones.com/2014 /03/approach/.

10. Blue Zones, "Blue Zones Project Home," https://info.bluezonesproject .com/home.

11. Dan Buettner, "Micro Nudges: A Systems Approach to Health," *American Journal of Health Promotion* 35, no. 4 (2021): 593–96, doi: 10.1177/08901171211 002328d.

12. Erin Hassanzadeh, "A Look Inside the United States' First-Ever Certified Blue Zone Located in Minnesota," CBS News, Dec. 1, 2023, https://www.cbsnews .com/minnesota/news/a-look-inside-the-united-states-first-ever-certified-blue -zone-located-in-minnesota/.

13. Blue Zones, "Albert Lea, MN: A Blue Zones Project Case Study," https:// cdn2.hubspot.net/hubfs/217817/BZP_AlbertLea_CaseStudy_102618.pdf.

14. Landscape Performance Series, "Cheonggyecheon Stream Restoration Project," https://www.landscapeperformance.org/case-study-briefs/cheonggyecheon -stream-restoration-project.

15. City of Melbourne, "Urban Forest Strategy: Making a Great City Greener 2012–2032," https://www.melbourne.vic.gov.au/urban-forest-strategy; Martin Hartigan et al., "Developing a Metropolitan-Wide Urban Forest Strategy for a Large, Expanding and Densifying Capital City: Lessons from Melbourne, Australia," *Land* 10, no. 8 (2021): 809, doi: 10.3390/land10080809.

16. University of California Davis Health, "Health and Place: A Green Prescription," https://health.ucdavis.edu/media-resources/chpr/documents/pdfs /PPPG/health-place-green-prescription.pdf.

17. Michelle C. Kondo et al., "Health Impact Assessment of Philadelphia's 2025 Tree Canopy Cover Goals," *Lancet Planetary Health* 4, no. 4 (2020): e149–e157, doi: 10.1016/S2542-5196(20)30058-9.

18. ECOBICI, "ECOBICI: Mexico City's Bike Sharing System," https:// ecobici.cdmx.gob.mx/en/.

19. ECOBICI, "Learn About the History of the Shared Bike System," https:// ecobici.cdmx.gob.mx/en/learn-about-the-history-of-the-shared-bike-system/.

20. LSE Latin America and Caribbean Centre, "What Can the Rest of the World Learn from Mexico City's ECOBICI Bike-Sharing Scheme?" https:// blogs.lse.ac.uk/latamcaribbean/2017/12/20/what-can-the-rest-of-the-world -learn-from-mexico-citys-ecobici-bike-sharing-scheme/.

21. Texas Health Resources, "Blue Zones Project Fort Worth," in *Community Responsibility Report 2021*, https://www.texashealth.org/responsibility-2021/Our -Communities/Blue-Zones-Project-Fort-Worth.

22. Blue Zones, "Blue Zones Project Results," https://info.bluezonesproject .com/results.

23. Blue Zones, "Fort Worth, TX: A Certified Blue Zones Community," https://cdn2.hubspot.net/hubfs/217817/National/BZP_ForthWorthBook_04 _PrintReady-Pages-compressed.pdf.

24. Tatiana Andreyeva et al., "Outcomes Following Taxation of Sugar-Sweetened Beverages: A Systematic Review and Meta-Analysis," *JAMA Network Open* 5, no. 6 (2022): e2215276, doi: 10.1001/jamanetworkopen.2022.15276.

25. City of Philadelphia, Philadelphia Beverage Tax (PBT), https://www.phila .gov/services/payments-assistance-taxes/taxes/business-taxes/business-taxes-by -type/philadelphia-beverage-tax-pbt/.

26. Jennifer Falbe et al., "Implementation of the First U.S. Sugar-Sweetened Beverage Tax in Berkeley, CA, 2015–2019," *American Journal of Public Health* 110, no. 9 (2020): 1429–37, doi: 10.2105/AJPH.2020.305795.

· 27. Matthew M. Lee et al., "Sugar-Sweetened Beverage Consumption 3 Years After the Berkeley, California, Sugar-Sweetened Beverage Tax," *American Journal of Public Health* 109, no. 4 (2019): 637–39, doi: 10.2105/AJPH.2019.304971; Joshua Petimar et al., "Sustained Impact of the Philadelphia Beverage Tax on Beverage Prices and Sales over 2 Years," *American Journal of Preventive Medicine* 62, no. 6 (2022): 921–29, doi: 10.1016/j.amepre.2021.12.012.

28. Kaitlyn Levinson, "Flat, Falling Soda Tax Revenues Have Both Positive and Negative Impact," City & State Pennsylvania, Oct. 8, 2024, https://www.city andstatepa.com/policy/2024/10/flat-falling-soda-tax-revenues-have-both-positive -and-negative-impact/400126/.

29. National Center for Statistics and Analysis, *Seat Belt Use in 2020—Use Rates in the States and Territories*, Traffic Safety Facts Crash Stats, Report No. DOT HS 813 109, National Highway Traffic Safety Administration, Apr. 2021, https://www.ktsro.org/files/Traffic-Facts-NHTSA-Seatbelt-Use-2020.pdf.

30. National Highway Traffic Safety Administration, "Seat Belts," https:// www.nhtsa.gov/vehicle-safety/seat-belts.

31. Feng J. He and Graham A. MacGregor, "A Comprehensive Review on Salt and Health and Current Experience of Worldwide Salt Reduction Programmes," *Journal of Human Hypertension* 23, no. 6 (2009): 363–84, doi: 10.1038/jhh.2008 .144; Pekka Puska and Paresh Jaini, "The North Karelia Project: Prevention of Cardiovascular Disease in Finland Through Population-Based Lifestyle

Interventions," *American Journal of Lifestyle Medicine* 14, no. 5 (2020): 495–99, doi: 10.1177/1559827620910981.

32. Pirjo Pietinen et al., "Labelling the Salt Content in Foods: A Useful Tool in Reducing Sodium Intake in Finland," *Public Health Nutrition* 11, no. 4 (2007): 335–40, doi: 10.1017/S1368980007000249.

33. Tiina Laatikainen et al., "Sodium in the Finnish Diet: 20-Year Trends in Urinary Sodium Excretion Among the Adult Population," *European Journal of Clinical Nutrition* 60, no. 8 (2006): 965–70, doi: 10.1038/sj.ejcn.1602406; Institute of Medicine (US) Committee on Strategies to Reduce Sodium Intake, Jeffrey E. Henney, Claire L. Taylor, and Carl S. Boon, eds., *Strategies to Reduce Sodium Intake in the United States* (Washington, DC: National Academies Press, 2010).

34. World Economic Forum, "50 Years of Ciclovía: Open Streets Cycling Cars," Nov. 2024, https://www.weforum.org/stories/2024/11/50-years-ciclovia-open-streets-cycling-cars/.

35. Eliza Barclay, "Bogotá Closes Its Roads Every Sunday. Now Everyone Wants to Do It," *Vox*, July 30, 2017, https://www.vox.com/2016/10/9/13017282/bogota-ciclovia-open-streets.

36. Costa Rica Immigrant Experts, "Costa Rica's Blue Zone: The Secrets of Longevity," https://crie.cr/about-the-blue-zone-in-costa-rica/.

37. Magdalini Kreouzi, Nikolaos Theodorakis, and Constantina Constantinou, "Lessons Learned from Blue Zones, Lifestyle Medicine Pillars and Beyond: An Update on the Contributions of Behavior and Genetics to Wellbeing and Longevity," *American Journal of Lifestyle Medicine* 18, no. 6 (2022): 750–65, doi:10.1177/15598276221118494.

38. Blue Zones, "Fort Worth, TX, Is Getting Healthier While Rest of Country Is Getting Sicker," Dec. 2018, https://www.bluezones.com/2018/12/fort-worth-tx-is-getting-healthier-while-rest-of-country-is-getting-sicker/.

39. Beach Cities Health District, "Healthy Living Programs," https://www.bchd.org/bzp.

40. Westside Health Authority, "Good Neighbor Campaign," https://gnc.healthauthority.org.

41. Australian Men's Sheds Association, "Australian Men's Sheds Association: Shoulder to Shoulder," https://mensshed.org.

42. Aisling McGrath et al., "Sheds for Life: Health and Wellbeing Outcomes of a Tailored Community-Based Health Promotion Initiative for Men's Sheds in Ireland," *BMC Public Health* 22, no. 1 (2022): 1590, doi: 10.1186/s12889-022-13964-6; Danielle Kelly et al., "Men's Sheds: A Conceptual Exploration of the Causal Pathways for Health and Well-Being," *Health & Social Care Community* 27, no. 5 (2019): 1147–57, doi: 10.1111/hsc.12765.

43. Danielle Kelly and Artur Steiner, "The Impact of Community Men's Sheds on the Physical Health of Their Users," *Health & Place* 71 (2021): 102649, doi: 10.1016/j.healthplace.2021.102649.

44. Saint Paul, Minnesota, Mayor's Office, https://www.stpaul.gov/departments/mayors-office.

Index